# I Can Speak Medical!

# I Can Speak Medical!

a concise guide to the
language of
medicine

by
Barbara E. Geary, BS, MA

*To your health!*
*Barbara E. Geary*

Epigraph Books
Rhinebeck, New York

Cover and book design by Colin Rolfe.
Cover art by Connor Malley.

ISBN: 978-1-944037-23-9
Library of Congress Control Number: 2016938822

Printed in the United States of America.

Epigraph Books
22 East Market Street, Suite 304
Rhinebeck, NY 12572
(845) 876-4861
www.epigraphps.com

# Table of Contents

# Introduction

*"No knowledge of a science can be properly acquired until the terminology of that science is mastered."*
—Spencer Trotter, Swarthmore College (1888–1926)

The purpose of this book is to make learning the language of medicine as simple and as much fun as possible—medspeak made accessible.

How did you learn to read? Was it while watching *Sesame Street*? Back in my day, it was by reading the Dick and Jane series. Those little books opened the whole big world of reading for me. This book can open for you the world of the language of medicine, or medspeak.

Knowledge of this language is essential for those preparing to become nurses and nurse aides, physicians, medical assistants, acupuncturists, dentists, dental hygienists, physical, and occupational therapists as well as health educators, massage therapists, medical billing specialists, insurance claim processors, pharmacists, and radiology professionals. Knowledge of the language of medicine assists those in related fields such as biomedical engineering, health information management, medical law practices, technical writers—well, the list could go on.

The field of healthcare is moving from a patriarchal "doctor knows best" approach to a participatory partnership characterized by informed choices and shared decision-making based on a person's goals, values, and where they are in life. Perhaps you have been a patient in a hospital or a parent concerned about a sick child. Perhaps you have accompanied an elderly relative on an office visit to their primary care practitioner. Perhaps in these situations you have wished that you knew more about what was being spoken around you, that you could penetrate the mystique shrouding very important information. Maybe you have searched the internet for information to help you to be proactive in maintaining or improving your own health and well-being and found that expanding your medical vocabulary would be useful. Learning the information presented here can be empowering, allowing you to participate more fully in your own health plan or that of a dependent.

Whatever your motivation for learning how to "speak medical," welcome! Chapter One lays out the basic fundamentals and guidelines. Chapters Two through Eleven cover vocabulary specific to the various body systems. Chapter Twelve contains some helpful tidbits, and the final chapter ends on a playful note.

Stories help you to remember, and I am a storyteller. Sometimes in this book it is a story about the word's history—its etymology. Sometimes it is a story from my nursing past, or a story a former student has shared. Along the way, I share mnemonics, tips to help you remember.

Sometimes that aid is a related word you already know. There is potential here for broadening your general vocabulary. Former students have told me that they will never look at words in the same way again.

As well as being a storyteller, I am a teacher. My educational credentials include a Bachelor of Science degree with a major in Nursing and a Master of Arts in Organization Development, a program that included a component on adult education.

In my work life as a registered professional nurse, I have held positions as varied as psychiatric staff nurse and nurse recruiter—one of the first in the United States. The continuing thread throughout my career, however, has been education. I have held positions in staff development in psychiatric as well as general hospital settings. I established a continuing education program for a professional nurses' association when the membership numbered over four thousand nurses. For a decade I taught an introduction to medical vocabulary at North Seattle College in Seattle, WA, where I designed and implemented the online version of the course.

P.S. Those Latin classes in high school have really paid off.

# Chapter One
## Building the Foundation

*"They do certainly give very strange, and newfangled, names to diseases."*
—Plato (c. 428–c. 348 BCE)

### Historical Roots

Let's begin with the origins of the language of Western medicine. Note that I have differentiated between Western medicine and other medical traditions. We will not be delving into the terms found in the rich heritages of such traditions as the Ayurvedic from India or the Chinese with its moxibustion, acupuncture, and energy meridians.

Most Western medical terms come from Latin or Greek roots. Hippocrates, a Greek physician who lived from c. 460 to c. 370 BCE, is known as the father of Western medicine. Some medical words he used are still in use today. The list includes apoplexy, hypochondria, dysentery, ophthalmia, epilepsy, and asthma.

The gods and goddesses of Greece and Rome are a historical source of medical terms. The following listing is a sampling of deities whose names we still remember through daily usage in medical settings, and elsewhere around the world. An example of a current related word is in **bold**.

Hygeia (daughter of Aesculapius, god of the healing arts) was the Greek goddess of health; **hygiene**.

Salus was the Roman goddess of health. *Salus* is the Latin word for health, welfare, safety; **salutation**.

Panacea, whose name is from the Greek meaning remedy or cure-all, was another daughter of Aesculapius; **panacea**.

Eos was the Greek goddess of the dawn; **eosinophyl**.

Iris was the goddess of the rainbow; **iris** as in the eye.

Hypnos was the Greek god of sleep; **hypnosis** literally means a condition of sleep.

Thanatos, Greek god of death, was Hypnos's twin brother; **euthanasia** literally indicates a gentle, easy death.

Somnus was the Roman god of sleep; **insomnia**.

Mnemosyne was the goddess of memory; **amnesia**.

Morpheus (the son of Hypnos) was known as the bringer of dreams; **morphine**.

Arachne was a mortal weaver who had the temerity to challenge the goddess Athena and was changed into a spider; **arachnophobia**.

Echo was a nymph attendant to the goddess Hera. She was so talkative that she was denied the power of speech, except to repeat what others said. She pined away to nothing but an answering voice; **echocardiogram**.

Priapus (son of Dionysus, who is associated with wine and revelry, and Aphrodite, Greek goddess of love) was the god of fertility and male generative power, the erect penis; **priapism**.

Genetyllis was the protectress of births and prayed to for problems of infertility; **genitalia**.

From these ancient roots to words so recently coined that they are heard only in the most esoteric of research facilities, the language of Western medicine is a living language: dynamic, fluid, yet full of history.

## Meanings Change

The meanings of words often change over time. One example would be the use of the word "broadcast." This word is an agricultural term for casting seed by hand. With the advent of the wireless telegraph in 1903, the word became associated with the transmitting of sound. Today both usages continue, but the historical connection is secondary. A medical example of a word that has changed in meaning is the word **hysteria**. A condition of the uterus. Early forebears in medicine thought that an empty, discontented uterus (belonging to a woman who was not pregnant) led to hysteria. This belief did not stand the test of time; we now know and acknowledge that both males and females are capable of emotional instability or excess.

## Some Basic Guidelines

Many medical terms can be broken down into component parts. These parts are the **word root**, **prefix**, and **suffix**. Breaking these terms down into their component parts helps to determine their meaning. An example is **cardiology**. This word is composed of the word root **cardi** (meaning heart) and the suffix **–logy** (meaning science or study of). Cardiology literally means the study of the heart.

Words that look complex are often the simplest because they can be broken down into these smaller parts. Let's look at **esophagogastroduodenoscopy**. The suffix **scopy** refers to a visual examination, **esophag** is the esophagus, **gastr** is the stomach, and **duoden** refers to the duodenum. So, taken all together, we have the diagnostic procedure that involves the insertion of an instrument to visually examine the esophagus, the stomach, and right through to the duodenum. Soon you will have the tools to decode words like this one. Saying this word without twisting your tongue all round—well, that's another challenge!

By contrast to decodable terms, there are terms that cannot be broken into parts. An example of such a word is **angina**. Angina comes from the Greek meaning strangling, which describes the characteristic pain of **angina pectoris**. Angina cannot be broken down into component parts; it has no prefix or suffix. You must just memorize such terms as one would when learning the irregular verbs of another language.

**Eponyms** are common to the medical language. The word "eponym" comes from the Greek *eponymos,* which means to be based upon someone's name. (**Epi** means upon and **nym** is name.) Some common examples of medical eponyms are:

• Parkinson's disease, after James Parkinson

• Alzheimer's dementia, after Alois Alzheimer
• Epstein-Barr virus, after Michael A. Epstein and Yvonne M. Barr
• Apgar's score, after Virginia Apgar
• Caesarean section, after the manner of Julius Caesar's birth (according to legend)

**Abbreviations** and **acronyms** are common to this language. BP is short for blood pressure and TPR stands for temperature, pulse, and respirations—the vital signs. CAD is coronary artery disease. (Computer-aided design is another field.) The abbreviation TLC can stand for a number of things such as thin-layer chromatography and total lung capacity. In nursing school, I learned another meaning that is so important to remember in the technical world of medicine: tender loving care.

In an **acronym** (**acr/o** means extremity or height, and **nym** means name), the initial letter or letters of the words in a name or term are combined. LASER is an acronym that stands for light amplification by stimulated emission of radiation.

### Four Word Parts

Using the word **pericardium** as our example, let's identify the word parts.

1. **Word root**  cardi
2. **Combining vowel**  o
3. **Prefix**  peri
4. **Suffix**  um

Note: The **combining form** is the word root and combining vowel taken together: **cardi/o.**

That's it!

Now, let's take a closer look at each of these components.

## Word Roots

A **word root** is the constant foundation and core of a medical term. All medical terms have one or more roots. A root can appear anywhere in the term. It can start the word without becoming a prefix. It can end the term without becoming a suffix. An example is **pneumothorax**. Both **pneum** and **thorax** are word roots. The letter **o** is a combining vowel.

## Combining Vowels

A **combining vowel** is also called a **connective vowel**. It is usually an **o** but can be an **i,** as in calcipenia, a **u**, as in virulent, or an **e**, as in cholecystectomy.

Why use a combining vowel? Whatever purpose does it serve? Good questions.

There are two guidelines for using combining vowels:

When connecting a word root and a suffix, a combining vowel is usually not used if the suffix begins with a vowel, as in peri cardi um not peri cardi o um. If the suffix begins with a consonant, generally the combining vowel is used, as in cardi o logy. The only reason I have ever seen for this guideline is to provide ease in pronunciation. The word flows more easily.

When connecting two word roots, a combining vowel is usually used even if vowels are present at the junction. An example is <u>gastr o enter o logy</u>.

The format used thenceforth to indicate a combining vowel used with a word root is: **word root/combining vowel,** as in **prostat/o**.

## Prefixes

A **prefix** precedes a root to change its meaning. Prefixes never require a combining vowel. An occasional medical term can have two prefixes. A prefix always appears at the beginning of the word. The clue here is **pre-**, which means before, earlier, prior, in front of. Not every medical term has a prefix.

## Suffixes

A **suffix** is attached to the end of a word root or combining form. A suffix changes the meaning of the word. If the suffix begins with a consonant, it follows a combining vowel. If the suffix begins with a vowel, no combining vowel is needed. A few medical terms have two suffixes. Not every medical term has a suffix.

That's it for technicalities! We can now grow some words. Changing only the suffix and keeping the word root constant, let's see how quickly your medical vocabulary can grow:

**arthr/o**   Joint.
**arthr/itis**   Inflammation of a joint.
**arthr/o/pathy**   Disease of a joint.
**arthr/o/scopy**   Visual examination of a joint.
**arthr/o/tomy**   Incision into a joint.
**arthr/o/plasty**   Surgical repair of a joint.
**arthr/algia**   Pain in a joint.

## Defining Terms

Note the definitions listed above. When defining a medical term, one starts with the **suffix**. One usually goes next to the **prefix**, if there is one, and then to the **word root**. Examples in addition to the list above are: **cardi/o/logy,** which is the study of the heart, and **macro/thromb/o/ cyt/o/penia,** which is a deficiency of large platelets found in the blood.

## Study Aids

There is nothing like repetition to help you learn new vocabulary words.

• Flash cards are a valuable study aid. Over my years of teaching, successful students repeatedly mentioned the indispensability of flash cards. Start with a 3x5 card. On one side, write the vocabulary word. On the other side, write the definition. There are flash cards online, or you can buy a set ready printed, but there is no substitute for actually writing the words out. Repetition creates an image in the brain and is good spelling practice. If the cards are kept handy, they can be referred to in a spare moment: standing in line, waiting for a bus, soaking in a tub.

• Say the words aloud.

• Have someone quiz you. Ask another person to give you a term so that you can respond with the definition. Then switch.

• Work without your flash cards. Write out vocabulary words that come to mind.

• Create your own mnemonics. I have suggested some mnemonics in this book to get you started.

# Chapter Two
## The Integumentary System

*"You're in pretty good shape for the shape you are in."*
—Dr. Seuss (1904–1991)

### Introduction

Let's start with the system that includes the most obvious components of our body: the skin, hair, and nails. These elements can be seen, touched, and smelled, and are familiar to us in ways that our inner parts are not.

The word "integumentary" comes to us from the Latin word *tegere*, meaning to cover, which is what the skin does so effectively. It is the largest organ of the body and the major component of the integumentary system. More minor coverage is provided by the hair (yes, with some people having more coverage than others) and the nails. The oil, or sebaceous, glands and the sweat, or sudoriferous, glands complete the inventory of the integumentary system.

## Function

The integumentary system, and particularly the skin, its major component, is charged with, well, holding us together. To this is added the responsibility of protection. This system protects underlying tissues from invasions of microbes. (Yes, they are out there—and out to get you!) It also protects those tissues from drying out and from harmful light rays. Add to this the help it provides in regulating body temperature. And its service as a sense organ (for the sense of touch). As well, this system assists in the elimination of waste via sweat and plays a role in the production of vitamin D.

# Key Vocabulary
## Skin

There are two primary combining forms meaning skin: **derm/o** or **dermat/o** and **cutane/o**.

1. **Derm/o** or **dermat/o**, coming from the Greek *derma*, translates to skin, hide, leather. Examples:

**derm/al**  Pertaining to the skin.

**dermat/o/logist**  One who has made a study of and specializes in the skin.

**hypo/derm/ic**  Pertaining to below the skin.

**intra/derm/al**  Pertaining to between the layers of the skin.

**dermat/itis**  Inflammation of the skin.

**erythr/o/derma**  Reddened skin.

**leuk/o/derma**  Abnormally white skin.

**pachy/derma**  Thickened skin.

**epi/derm/o/myc/osis** A condition involving a fungus on the skin.

*2.* **Cutane/o** is from the Latin *cutis,* meaning skin. Examples:
  **cutane/ous**   Pertaining to the skin.
  **sub/cutane/ous**   Pertaining to under the skin.

A lesser-used word for skin, "pelt," is of uncertain origin but tied to the Latin *pellis* or *pellicula*. It is more commonly used for the skin of an animal with the fur still on it. However, the derivative word **pellagra** is heard in medical circles and indicates a chronic disease characterized by skin eruptions. There is also the word **erysipelas**, which literally refers to red skin and is the name of a skin infection. Some non-medical derivatives are "pellicle," which means a thin skin, and in fashion a "pelisse," which refers to a lady's or child's cloak reaching to the ankles, quite effectively covering the person wearing it.

There is yet another word for skin: **corium**. It is found in the word **excoriate**, which literally means to remove the skin from. In medspeak, it means to abrade, scrape, or chafe. In other settings, it is used to mean a severe censuring or criticizing, to lambast, or to slam someone.

### Hair

Hair also has two common combining forms: **pil/o** or **pil/i** and **trich/o**.

1. **Pil/o** or **pil/i** derives from the Latin *pilus,* meaning hair. Examples:
  **pil/i/form**   Hairlike (*forma* means shape).
  **pil/o/sity**   Having or being covered with hair; hairiness.
  **de/pil/atory**   A substance used to remove unwanted hair.

**pil/o/nid/al**   A painful cyst containing hair located between the buttocks, in the butt crack (*nidus* is Latin for nest)

2. **Trich/o** is from the Greek meaning hair. Examples:
   **trich/o/logy**  The study of hair, its care and treatment.
   **trich/o/gen**  An agent that stimulates hair growth.
   **trich/o/megaly**  Long, coarse eyebrows.
   **trich/o/pathy**  Disease conditions of hair.
   **trich/o/phobia**  An abnormal dread of hair or of touching it.
   **trich/o/phagia**  The habit of eating hair.
   **trich/o/myc/osis**  Any disease of the hair caused by a fungus.

A less common combining form is **hirsut/o**, which is found in **hirsutism**, a condition of excessive growth of hair or the presence of hair in unusual places. *Hirsutus* is the Latin word for shaggy. A former student looking for a way to remember this word came up with the mnemonic hairsuit/ hirsute. Good job!

Let's not neglect that special soft, downy hair that covers a fetus and sometimes the newborn: **lanugo** from the Latin meaning down.

### Nails

Perhaps you've noticed a pattern: two combining forms meaning hair, two common ones meaning skin, and in each case one comes from the Latin and one from Greek lineage. The nails are no exception. Their two combining forms are **onych/o** and **ungu/o**.

1. **Onych/o** derives from the Greek *onyx*, which means nail. Examples:

>**ep/onych/ium**   Literally, the structure or tissue above or on the nail; also called the cuticle.
>
>**onych/o/crypt/osis**   Literally, the condition of a hidden nail; an in-grown nail.
>
>**onych/o/malacia**   The softening of a nail.
>
>**onych/o/myc/osis**   The condition of a nail caused by a fungus.
>
>**onych/o/phagia**   Literally, to eat the nail; in common usage, a nail-biter.
>
>**onych/ectomy**   The surgical removal or resection of a nail.

2. **Ungu/o** comes to us from the Latin *unguis*. Example:

>**ungu/al**   Pertaining to or resembling the nail.

## Glands

The skin, the hair, the nails, and now the vocabulary associated with the glands.

The oil, or sebaceous, glands and the sweat, or sudoriferous, glands are exocrine glands. The **ex-** in **exocrine** means out or away from, and **-crine** means to secrete. **Exo/crine** glands secrete out of the body as opposed to **endo/crine** glands, which secrete within the body. We will meet up with some endocrine glands in a later chapter. Meanwhile, the combining form for gland is **aden/o** as in **adenoids**, which literally means to resemble (**-oid**) a gland.

Now, let's do some more translation.

**Sebace/ous** comes from the Latin meaning wax or tallow. The combining form is **seb/o** or **sebace/o** for this term indicating the oil glands.

There are three combining forms for the sweat glands: **sudor/i** and **diaphor/o**, and **hidr/o**.

*Sudor* is a Latin word for sweat and **sudor/i/fer/ous** means to convey or produce (**fer**) sweat.

1. Besides *sudor*, there is another combining form from Latin meaning sweat: **hidr/o**. Examples:
> **hyper/hidr/osis**   A condition in which the production of sweat is excessive. Your palms may be always moist, even when you are not nervous, for example. Night sweats are referred to as **sleep hyper/hidr/osis**.
> **an/hidr/osis**  The condition when no sweat is produced.
> **hidr/aden/itis**   Referring to the inflammation of a sweat gland.

2. The Greek combining form for sweat is **diaphor/o**, which literally means to carry or bear (**phor**) through or complete (**dia**).

**Diaphor/esis** is profuse sweating and is normally experienced after physical exercise or on hot, humid days, or during a menopausal hot flash. When I was in nursing school we wore diaphoresis shirts, not sweatshirts.

### Additional Vocabulary

Now, let's become acquainted with some other combining forms, as well as words that do not break down into parts, that are used in association with the integumentary system. We will start with comparing the differences of meaning of the following word roots: **aut/o**, **heter/o**, and **hom/o**.

1. **Aut/o** refers to one's self, as in autobiography, a story of one's own life (bio). Or as in automobile, a vehicle in which one can move around on one's own and not wait for an omnibus, which provides transportation for all (*omni* is Latin for all.) Over the years, the prefix has been dropped, but we still ride the bus all around the town. In a medical and integumentary context, we might see these combining forms used with graft, as in a skin graft. If the source of the graft is one's own body, then the graft is called an **auto/ graft** or **auto/logous**, or a **dermat/o/auto/plasty**.

2. If the donor and recipient are different people, the procedure is called a **dermat/o/heter/o/plasty** or an **allo/ graft**. Both **all/o** and **heter/o** mean different or another.

3. If the procedure involves a donor and recipient from different species, as when putting a bovine valve in a human heart, the term used is **heter/o/graft** or **xen/o/ graft**. **Xen/o** means strange or foreign. If the donor is from the same species as the recipient, the term used is **homo/ graft**. **Hom/o** means same. (This usage is from the Greek; the Latin word part *homo-* means mankind.)

Now let's learn more words commonly used in the integumentary system.

**Cyan/o** is from the Greek *kyanos*, meaning blue. **Cyan/osis**, literally a condition of blueness, is the skin discoloration indicating reduced oxygen in the blood.

**Elast/o** may be familiar because of our word "elastic," which means capable of being stretched and then returning to the original state; the elasticity of the skin diminishes as one grows older.

**Erythr/o** is from the Greek *erythros* which means red. **Eryth/ema** is a general term referring to redness of the skin.

**Fibr/o** means just what it looks like: fiber, as in **fibr/ous** tissues.

**Kerat/o** comes from the Greek *keras*, meaning horn. **Kerat/o** and **scler/o** share a sense of hardness. **Keratin** is a tough, horny protein found in the dead outer layer of skin, nails, and hair. **Scler/o/derma** literally means hard skin.

**Lei/o** means smooth and has done so since the Romans used the word *leios* to describe a baby's bottom. The Greeks used the same word. But if you say **lei/o/derm/ia** to a medical practitioner, they will interpret it as a skin condition in which the skin is abnormally smooth and glossy.

**Leuk/o** is from the Greek *leukos*, meaning white. **Leuk/o/cytes**, white blood cells, and **leuk/emia**, which literally translates as a condition of white blood (**-emia**) are familiar uses of the combining form. A condition of the skin involving this combining form is **leuk/o/derma**, which is another name for **vitiligo**. Vitiligo is characterized by patches of abnormally light-colored skin.

**Lip/o**, **steat/o**, and **adip/o** are three combining forms meaning fat. **Lipids**, **lip/o/suction**, **steat/o/rrhea**, and **adip/ose** tissue are examples of their use.

**Melan/o** is from the Greek *melas*, meaning black or dark. **Melanin** is the pigment (from the Latin meaning paint, by the way) produced by **melan/o/cytes**. And **melan/omas** (**-oma** means tumor or mass) are familiar as skin cancer.

**Pachy/o** means thick, large and massive; **pachyderm** means thick skinned.

**Rhytid/o** brings to mind cosmeticians and plastic surgeons for this combining form comes from the Greek *rhytis*, meaning wrinkle. Facelifts in medspeak are **rhytid/ectomies** (**-ectomy** means to surgically remove, excise, or resection). The term **rhytid/o/plasty** also applied: **-plasty** means to surgically repair. If you think you see "plastic" in that suffix, you are correct. The Greek root is *plassein* and means to form, shape, or mold.

**Sarc/o** means flesh. You may have seen the root in sarcophagus, a type of stone used for coffins and another word for a casket or coffin. It literally means flesh-eating and refers to the supposed action of the stone on decomposing bodies. A medical condition containing this combining form is **sarc/oid/osis**. Another is **sarc/o/lysis**, a condition marked by the decomposition, or break-down, of soft tissues or flesh. The suffix **-lysis** means breakdown, dissolving, or loosening. To lyse is to destroy. Think Lysol.

## Dermatology

"Dermatology" is the word used when speaking of the study of the skin and its diseases. Below you will find some of the more common words and word roots which name conditions, symptoms, or signs.

**Abras/o** may be familiar as **abrasion**. It comes from the Latin meaning to scrape, and that is what an abrasion is, scraped skin.

**Abscess** comes from the Latin *ab-*, away from, and the infinitive *cedere*, meaning to go. An abscess is a painful, inflamed area filled with pus. Now, the combining form for pus is **py/o**; for inflammation we generally use the suffix **-itis** and for pain, **-algia**. None of these word parts is evident here. How did "to go away from" become the name of this nasty sore? Hippocrates' theory of bodily humors tells us that the humors go from the body through the pus. (In the chapter on the circulatory systems we will learn a bit more about this interesting theory.)

**Albinism** is a genetic condition marked by partial or total absence of melanin in the skin.

**Alopecia** originally referred to a mangy fox but has come to mean a lack of scalp hair, or baldness. Fascinating, the journey words take over time.

**Carbuncle** is another word that has had an intriguing journey. Originally it meant fiery jewel or red gem and referred to rubies, garnets, and such. Later, it was used to refer to an abscess in which two or more boils (**furuncles**) had merged. I remember seeing only one carbuncle in my life and that was when I was a young child: it was on the back of my grandfather's neck. Nasty-looking thing it was.

**Carcin/o** is a familiar combining form. It comes from the Greek meaning crab, the mascot or symbol of the Zodiacal sign Cancer. **Carcin/o/genic**, pertaining to that which has the potential to cause cancer, is an example of the use of this combining form.

**Cicatrix** sounds like "sick of tricks" and means a scar.

**Comedo** is commonly called a blackhead.

**Contusion** is another word for a bruise.

**Crypt/o** comes to us from the Greek *kryptos*, which means hidden, concealed or secret. You will notice as we go along that a Greek word spelled with a 'k' is often spelled with a 'c' in English. There was no letter 'c' in the Greek language, just the 'k'. Hence, crypt/o and *kryptos*. Superman fans will see a resemblance to the hero's home planet, Krypton, and Kryptonite, which has the power to do him in. Chemistry students will see the gas, krypton. And some may see the field of study: cryptozoology: the study of unknown, legendary or extinct animals whose existence or survival is disputed or unsubstantiated.

**Debridement** is French, literally meaning a debridling, and is the cleansing of a wound: the removing of foreign material and dead or damaged tissue. When my sister was a little girl, she fell out of our 1936 Plymouth onto the berm of the road. Her body slid along the cinders from the velocity. In the Emergency Room, she had multiple abrasions which needed to be cleaned, or debrided.

**Decubitus ulcer** is a pressure sore. The word decubitus comes to us from the Latin *de-*, meaning down, and *cubere*, to lie. This takes us back to the custom of Roman men to recline on their couches sipping wine and discussing the affairs of state. Too much wining and reclining on one's elbows leads to a breakdown of the skin, an ulcer. The word discubiture refers to a reclining posture assumed when dining. The Latin *cubitum* means elbow. The **antecubital** space is in front of the elbow, at the bend in the arm. **Ante-** means before. If you look again at the Latin *cubitum*, you will see the ancient unit of measure, the cubit, which brings us to cubicle - a space big enough to perhaps stand with elbows akimbo.

**Ichthy/o** means fish in the Greek; **ichthy/osis** is a condition marked by dry, scaly, fish-like skin.

**Jaundice** comes to us from the French and means 'yellow'. The condition is marked by a yellowish cast to the skin. The Latin word for jaundice is *icterus*, a word you may also see in medical settings.

**Keloid** comes from the Greek *kelis*, which means blemish. A keloid is a result of an overgrowth of scar tissue during the healing process. Those little cells so energetically, profusely, well, just overdoing it a bit.

**Laceration** comes from the Latin meaning ripping or tearing. A laceration is an irregular, rough or jagged tear of the skin.

**Necr/o** is another gift from the Greeks, *nekros*, meaning death. A **necroscopy** (**-scopy** means to make a visual examination) is another word for autopsy. And there we have aut/o again. An autopsy is the term generally used in the examination of human corpses while necropsy is generally reserved for animals.

**Onych/o/phagia** is a condition in which one bites one's nails, a nail-biter. The suffix **-phagia** is from the Greek *phagos* and means "eating." The combining form is **phag/o**.

**Pedicul/o** comes to us from the Latin *pediculus* which means louse. **Pedicul/osis** is a condition of an infestation with lice.

**Petechiae** (the singular is petechia) are tiny pinpoint hemorrhages into the skin which resemble little flea bites.

**Pruritus** simply means itching. Please note the spelling here! It is easy to confuse the suffix -itis with this 'us' ending. An **anti-pruritic** would be a treatment. **Anti-**, meaning against.

**Psoriasis** is a challenge for spellers. (The 'p' is silent.) You can recognize this condition of the skin when you see it because of its characteristic silvery scales covering red lesions.

**Purpura** is a rash of sites in which blood cells leak into the skin. Pinpoint purpura are called petechiae and larger ones are called **ecchymoses** (the singular being ecchymosis).

**Purulent** is the word meaning to form or contain pus.

**Py/o** comes to us from the Greek and means pus. **Pyo/rrhea** is a condition characterized by a flow or discharge of pus.

**Seps/o** is from the Greek *sepsis*, which has become an English word as well and is translated as rot or putrefaction. A **sept/ic** condition is a systemic inflammatory response to infection.

**Tinea** is medical-speak for ringworm, a fungal skin disease.

**Urticaria** is also known as hives. In Latin *urtica* means nettle.

**Verrucae** are skin lesions caused by the human papilloma virus (HPV) and are also known as warts.

**Xer/o** means dry. While spending time in the Southwest USA, one might become familiar with xeroscaping - a landscaping style which requires little water. Xeric, pertaining to dryness, is used when referring to something which requires only a small amount of water. And then there is Xerox. It is a copying process which uses dry ink. When it comes to medspeak, dry skin is known as **xer/o/derma**.

### Just a Few More for Good Measure...

A **macule** is flat, like a freckle while a **papule** is raised, coming as it does from the Latin meaning pimple.

A **vesicle** is a blister measuring less than 1 cm while a **bulla** is greater than 1 cm.

A **cyst** is a sac filled with fluid or semisolid material while a **nodule** is a solid lesion. The Latin *nodulus* means little knot.

**Plaque** is illustrated by dandruff.

**Pustules** are pimples containing pus.

**Wheals** are also known as welts.

Good job!

# Chapter Three
## The Musculoskeletal System

*"The patient must combat the disease along with the physician."*
—Hippocrates (c. 460–c. 370 BCE)

### Introduction

Just under the skin is the framework of our body, the **skeleton**. *Skeletos* is a Greek word meaning dried up, and back in the day, a *skeleton soma* referred to a dried-up body, parched and withered, a mummy. The word *soma* means body. Over the years, the word **skeleton** also took on the meaning of a bare outline, something reduced to minimum form. It is in this context that we speak of a skeleton crew, or a skeleton key, or the bony framework for our body. Skeletons in the closet? That's for another time and place! But what is an **ex/o/skeleton**? (Hint: **ex/o-** means from, out of, or outside.) Yes, the skeleton is on the outside in creatures such as the grasshopper, and takes the form of a shell in lobsters and crabs.

The human skeletal system is composed of bones, bone marrow, cartilage, joints, ligaments, synovial membrane, synovial fluid, and bursa.

The other focus of this chapter is the muscles of the body. Muscle in Latin is *musculus*, or little mouse. Some ancient scholar may have thought that the flexing of a muscle resembled the movements of a wee mouse. Or perhaps that some muscles looked mouse-like in form. From the Greek, the combining form is **my/o:** *mys* means both mouse and muscle. Now, no more will you have a cramp or a charley horse! You now can call it a **my/o/spasm**.

The components of the muscular system are the skeletal muscles (as opposed to the cardiac muscles) and the tendons.

**Function**

The skeletal part of the musculoskeletal system provides the framework for the body; it gives shape. It also supports and protects the internal organs. The joints work with the muscles, ligaments, and tendons to make possible the wide variety of body movements. This system provides for mineral storage, e.g. calcium and phosphorus. In the red bone marrow is found activity essential to blood formation (**hemat/o/poiesis**). And then there is the task of detoxification: the bones remove metals such as lead and radium from the blood, store them, and then slowly release them for excretion from the body.

The muscular system is all about movement, support, and heat production.

# Key Vocabulary
## Bone

There are two combining forms meaning bone: **oste/o** and **osse/o**.

1. The Greeks contributed the combining form **oste/o**. Examples:

**oste/o/cyte**   The suffix refers to a cell, so literally, this is a cell of a bone.

**oste/o/arthr/itis**   The degeneration of cartilage and bone in a joint.

**oste/o/por/osis**   A loss of bone density. This condition gradually changed my mother's height from 5'11" to around 5'6".

**oste/o/phytes**   Bone spurs. Calling them **osteophytes** doesn't help the pain or the limitation of movement caused by the spurs, but it shows that you can speak medical! The suffix **-phyte** comes to us from the Greek *phyton,* which means plant. **-Phyte** is used to mean both plant and abnormal growth, the latter being the case with bone spurs.

**osteo/malacia**   Pertaining to the softening of bone tissue.

**ost/ectomy**   The surgical removal or resection of a bone.

**oste/o/plasty**   The surgical repair of bone.

**oste/o/necr/osis**   The condition of dead bone; the word root **necr/o** means dead.

**oste/o/myel/itis**   The inflammation of bone and bone marrow.

**peri/oste/um**   The suffix **-um** signifies a noun meaning structure, tissue, or thing; the prefix **peri-** means around, so we have a tissue surrounding a bone.

2. The Romans contributed the combining Latin form **osse/o**. Examples:

**oss/ify**  To become bone tissue.

**ossi/fic/ation**  The process of turning into or becoming bone.

**oss/uary**  A depository for the bones of the dead.

**oss/icle**  From the Latin *ossiculum,* the word literally means a little bone but often specifically refers to the three **ossicles** in the ear. **Ossicle** is the diminutive of **osse.**

**ossi/form**  Resembling bone; the suffix **-form** refers to a resemblance or   taking the shape or form of.

**osse/ous**  Pertaining to bone or bonelike.

**osse/o/integr/ation**  The anchoring of prosthetic material into bone.

### Bone Marrow

The Greeks have contributed the combining form meaning marrow and spinal cord: **myel/o**. Examples:

**myel/o/dys/plasia**  Marked by defective formation of the spinal cord; **dys-** means abnormal, impaired or difficult, and **-plasia** means development or formation. It is also a **hematological** disease, a blood disorder involving the formation of blood cells in the bone marrow.

**myel/oma**  A tumor (**-oma** means tumor or mass) of the bone marrow.

### Cartilage

There are two combining forms meaning **cartilage: cartilag/o** and **chondr/o**.

1. The first, **cartilag/o**, comes directly to us from the Latin and means cartilage or gristle. Examples:

>**cartilag/inous** Pertaining to or consisting of cartilage.
>**cartilag/ini/fication** Cartilage formation; development of cartilage.

2. The Greek combining form is **chondr/o**. Examples:

>**chondr/oma** A tumor (**-oma** means tumor or mass) of cartilage tissue.
>**a/chondr/o/plasia** A lack of or abnormally slow development of bone  cartilage. The prefix **a-** or **an-** means no, not, without. The suffix **-plasia** m e a n s development, growth, formation, or shaping.
>**chondr/o/malacia** A softening of cartilage; **-malacia** means pertaining to softening.
>**chondro/blast** A cell that forms cartilage; an immature cartilage cell.
>**chondro/costal** Pertaining to rib cartilage; *costa* is Latin for rib.
>**chondro/dynia** Pain in the cartilage; **chondralgia** would also be correct: the  suffixes  **-algia**  and **-dynia** both mean pain.
>**chondro/tome** A device for cutting cartilage; **-tome** is an instrument to cut.

## Joints

There are two combining forms for joint: **articul/o** and **arthr/o**. The word joint comes from the Latin *junctus*, meaning united or connected.

1. If you know what an articulated vehicle is, you have a start on the Latin combining form for joint: **articul/o**.

An **articulation** is a joint. In dentistry, to **articulate** is to arrange teeth on a denture. Another usage is to articulate one's words, meaning to speak clearly and distinctly.

2. From the Greek, we get the combining form **arthr/o**. Examples:

>**arthr/itis**   Joint inflammation. In medieval times arthr/itis was known as "joint evil."
>**arthr/algia**   Literally, a painful joint; the suffix **-algia** means pain.
>**arthr/o/scopy**   The suffix **-scopy** refers to a visual examination, which in this case is of a joint.

### Ligaments

*Ligamentum* is the Latin for a tie or ligature, a binding. **Ligaments** connect one bone to another.

### Synovial Membrane and Fluid

**Synovial fluid** is an albuminous liquid that lubricates the joints; the **synovial membrane** provides a lining. Does the presence of **ov,** meaning egg (*ovum* in Latin), in the word **synovial** relate to the egg-white appearance of this fluid? Some have thought so.

### Bursa

A **bursa** is a small pouch or sac usually found near joints. It is lined with synovial membrane and filled with synovial fluid. From the Latin, *bursa* is a bag or purse. A bursar is a treasurer of a college or university, the one who carries the purse. Have you ever been reimbursed for your expenses? A purse of money was involved, figuratively if not literally.

Back to medical terms:

**burs/itis**   An inflammation of the **bursa**.

**burs/o/lith**   The presence of a stone (or **calculus**) in a bursa.

**burs/ectomy**   The surgical removal or resection of a bursa.

## Muscle

As noted in the introduction, the combining form for muscle is **my/o**. Examples:

**my/algia**   Pain in a muscle or muscles.

**my/o/cele**   A herniated muscle.

**my/o/rrhaphy**   The suturing of a muscle; the suffix **-rrhaphy** refers to suturing

## Tendons

Finally, we have the **tendons**: from the Greek, the combining form is **ten/o,** and in the Latin, the combining form is **tendin/o**. The Latin infinitive *tendere* means to stretch and is related to this word. Tendons connect muscles to bones. Examples:

**tend/o/lysis**   The process of freeing a tendon from adhesions; **-lysis** means to break down, separate, destroy, or loosen.

**tend/o/vagin/al**   Pertaining to a tendon and its sheath; *vagina* is the Latin word for sheath.

## Additional Vocabulary

You have an **acr/om/ion**. It is found, simply put, where the scapula articulates with the clavicle—or more simply, where your shoulder blade meets your collarbone. The word part **acr/o** means highest point or extremity. Think Acropolis, the highest point in the city, the acme. Or **acr/o/phobia**, the abnormal fear of high places. Then there is the acrobat, someone who works in high places. In acromion, **om/o** means shoulder; the suffix **-ion** means process.

**Ankyl/o** means crooked, bent, or stiff in the sense of fused; **ankyl/osis** is the immobility of a joint.

**Brachi/o** refers to the arm; the **brachioradialis** is a muscle in the forearm. In my online class, I used to ask students to contribute a word to the discussion forum using the word root **brachi**. One contribution I remember was "brachiate": a monkey brachiates from limb to limb in trees; a child brachiates or swings from hold to hold on—monkey bars.

You've heard of **carpal** tunnel syndrome. **Carp/o** means wrist; the **carp/al** tunnel carries nerves through the wrist.

Consider the hand: **chir/o** comes from the Greek; the Latin equivalent is **manu**. "Manuscript" and "chirography" are synonymous, both meaning a handwritten record or document. A chiropractor's treatment involves the manipulation or manual adjustment of bone position. Puts a different slant on "maneuver," doesn't it? And "manure." We think of "manure" as a noun, which it is, referring to dung, compost, fertilizer. But the word was once used as a verb in the sense of working or cultivating the soil with the hands.

The **clavicle** is more readily recognized by its common name, the collarbone. The source of this word is the Latin *clavis*, meaning key. Clavicle is the diminutive: little key. The English word "enclave" carries with it the sense of being enclosed, shut in, indeed locked in. A similar word is "conclave," the meeting or place where cardinals in the Roman Catholic Church gather to elect a pope. The word literally translates "with key." The cardinals gather together in a locked room until they conclude their task.

The Greek word for key is *kleis*, which gives us the medical term: **stern/o/cleid/o/ mastoid**, a muscle in the neck. Also, the name Cleopatra.

The **coccyx** was named by ancient Greek physicians. They saw a resemblance between the human coccyx, when viewed from the side, and the beak of the cuckoo bird. The word *kokkyx* is Greek for cuckoo bird. Another descriptive name for the coccyx is the tailbone.

**Cost/o** is the combining form for rib. A **cost/ectomy** refers to the surgical excision or resection of a rib.

**Cran/o** or **crani/o** means skull, as in **crani/um** or **crani/al**.

The **gluteus maximus** is the largest muscle in the body. Another name for this muscle is the buttock. Which segues to a story. When I was teaching, I got some of my best material from students. One day, before class had begun, a student approached me with a word that her boyfriend had used to describe her: "callipygian." She asked if I knew what it meant. I broke the word down into its component parts. Calli is the equivalent of the Greek *kalli,* which means beautiful. In Greece you greet one other with *kalimera* (good morning) or *kalispera* (good evening). The word "calligraphy" refers to beautiful writing. *Pygos* or *pyge* (in the Greek) means buttocks. He had just told her she had a shapely posterior! How nice...

To the moon, which also has a tie with buttocks in slang. Here, the term we are learning refers to the crescent moon. The **meniscus** is a crescent-shaped cartilage cushioning the knee. This word also refers to the curve in the upper surface of a liquid. **Lunula** is the Latin for little moon and can be found in the whitish crescent at the base of a fingernail and in the semilunar valve of the heart.

The Latin word *crepitus* means rattling, crackling, creaking. When this happens in an osteoarthritic knee, it is called **crepitation**. You may also hear **crepitations** when bones are broken or pneumonia is present in the lung.

**Kinesi/o** means motion. **Kinetics** relates to motion. **Dys/kinesia** means painful or difficult movement, while **brady/kinesia** pertains to extreme slowness of movement.

There are several –oids associated with the skeletal system. In the skull, we can find three of them. First, let's establish that the suffix -oid means resembling, having the appearance of. The **sphen/oid** bone (**sphen/o** means wedge) resembles a wedge or was thought to by those who named it. The **ethm/oid** (**ethm/o** means sieve) has tiny holes in it. The **mast/oid** (**mast/o** means breast) was thought to resemble the shape of a breast or nipple. Elsewhere in the skeleton, we have the **xiph/oid** process, composing the lower part of the sternum or breastbone; **xiph/o** means sword. **Styl/oid** means resembling a stylus or pointed instrument. **Styl/oid** processes can be found on some bones. Finally, there is the **hy/oid** bone, which comes from the Greek meaning shaped like the letter *u*. The **hy/oid** is found between the chin and the **thyr/oid**, a gland we will meet in a subsequent chapter.

**Patella** comes to us directly from the Latin and means kneecap.

---

Our fingers and toes are sometimes called **digits**. This word comes from the Latin *digitus*, meaning finger or toe. Digits also refer to numeric symbols. Counting on the fingers and toes, that makes sense. The foxglove plant, from the genus *digitalis* meaning finger-like, refers to the flower's thimble (fitting over a finger) shape. The medicine digitalis was originally extracted from the plant. Sometimes the fingers and toes are called **phalanges**. This word comes to us from the military. A *phalanx* (Latin/Roman) is a unit of heavily armed foot soldiers in close, deep ranks. Just think of your fingers and toes as rows of little soldiers. The plural of phalanx is **phalanges**.

A third combining form meaning a finger or toe is **dactyl/o**. **Poly/dactyly** means having more than the usual five fingers or toes. **Brachy/dactyly** describes unusually short fingers and toes. **Syn/dactyly** is the condition in which two or more digits are joined together—webbed, as it were. I have been told that this condition, also known as **sym/physis**, is a usual occurrence when one has lived in Seattle for over five years, due to the oceanic or maritime climate of that city.

---

*Rectus* is a Latin word meaning straight. The **rectum** is the straight section of the lower intestine that comes after the curves of the **sigm/oid** segment of the colon, which resembles the Greek letter carrying the *s* sound, the *sigma*. There are a number of muscles that bear this name: **rectus abdominis**, **rectus femoris**, the lateral **rectus** muscle of the eye, and those tiny muscles found at the base of each hair follicle, the **erector** muscles, which make our hair stand on end and give us goose bumps from fright or cold.

There is a depression in the **sphen/oid** bone of the skull in which one finds the pituitary gland. This depression is called the **sella turcica**, or Turkish saddle. What imagination that early anatomist displayed!

**Spondyl/o** is the word root meaning vertebra. It comes to us from the Greek. The Latin word root is **vertebr/o**. **Spondyl/o/listhesis** is more fun to say than to have as a diagnosis, since it involves the slippage of one vertebra forward on the one below it. The resulting compression on nerve roots causes pain.

### One More for Good Measure

It comes in handy when cuddling a baby or a lover. The word **nucha** or **nuque**, refers to the nape of the neck. Nibbling the nucha.

## Maladies and Unwellnesses

Sometimes a person has to have a limb amputated. While the word **amputation** is commonly known and understood, it is informative to know that it comes to us from the Latin meaning to cut or prune.

---

There are three terms which have to do with spinal alignment.

1. The first is **kyph/o**, which in Greek means crooked. **Kyph/osis** is the condition commonly referred to as humpback or hunchback. **Kypho/sis** can occur at any age, but is more common among older women when you may hear it called a "dowager's hump." A dowager is a widow who has inherited property or a title from her late husband, and, by extension, a dignified elderly woman.

2. The second term is **lord/o** (bending). **Lord/osis,** the condition of an anterior curvature of the lumbar spine, is commonly called swayback.

3. The third is **scoli/osis** (**scoli/o** means bent, stiff, crooked, or curved). It is a lateral curvature of the spine. Scoli/o comes from the Latin; the Greek is **ankyl/o**. **Ankyl/osis** refers to the stiffening of joints after injury or surgery. It can also mean the intentional fixation of separate bone parts to form one.

---

**Orth/o** means straight. **Orth/o/ped/ic** literally means pertaining to a straight child, **ped/o** coming from the Greek meaning child. The term originally was used in addressing parents and those others involved in child rearing. Later it came to refer to physicians and bones. In **orthodontia, dont/o** means teeth; therefore we have a condition (**-ia**) of straight teeth. Interestingly, "orthodox" literally means straight thinking. There have been wars fought over just whose thinking is straight and whose is heretical. In less heated situations than wars, orthodoxy is the conventional, the commonly accepted, the mainstream. But heretics are still accused of iconoclastic behavior. (Icon means image and the suffix **-clast** means to break.) Which leads us back to bones. **Oste/o/clasis** refers to the intentional breaking of a bone to correct a defect.

**Para/pleg/ia** is a condition of paralysis (**pleg**) of the lower half of the body and of both legs. In the original Greek, paraplegia referred to paralysis of one side of the body. The term **hemi/pleg/ia** is the word we use today to refer to paralysis of one vertical side of the body. And the prefix **para-**? It means alongside or near. Some familiar words using this prefix are: paramedical, paralegal, paratransit, paratrooper, parallel, and paradox.

Previously, we learned that **ped/o** comes from the Greek meaning child. This is still true; but just to confuse the issue, the Latin *pedis* means foot—as in "pedestrian" and "pedometer." The context will tell you whether **ped/o** means a child or a foot. In the Greek, it is **pod/o** that means foot. As in **podiatrist**, one who specializes in treatment of foot problems. Another example is "tripod," which literally means having three feet.

---

**Quadri-** is a prefix meaning four. Some relatively well-known words with this as their prefix are: **quadriceps** (**ceps** comes to us via **caput**, meaning head), quadrant (from the Latin for the fourth part), quadrilateral (pertaining to four sides; *latus* is Latin for side), and **quadr/i/pleg/ic** (**pleg** from the Greek meaning paralysis or palsy).

But did you ever connect the word quarantine with the **quadri-** words? It is a relative with an interesting history. The connection is with the number four, which has now become forty. *Quaranta* is Italian for forty. It was first used, I understand, in the Magna Carta as a word meaning a forty-day period during which a widow could legally stay in her deceased husband's house without the heirs to the property coming to hassle her. During the Black Plague in Europe, it came to mean the forty-day period in which a ship and its occupants were held in port to determine whether the passengers were free of disease. It has come to be synonymous with enforced isolation and can now be for any period of time. I have photos from my parents' and grandparents' day that show signs on doors of houses giving notice that the family living there was being kept in quarantine, perhaps for scarlet fever or diphtheria. I also remember enjoying the privilege of visiting with a woman who was a friend of my parents until her passing at age ninety-eight. She would tell me the story of how, at a time when her family was under quarantine, my parents would bring food, place it on the porch, and call out before leaving. It meant so much to them, she said, as there were some who were afraid to come close to the house. In medical-speak today quarantine is referred to as **isolation**.

---

Now to the combining form **tax/o.** The Greek *taxis* means arrangement, as in a certain order or coordination. A taxonomy has to do with scientific classification. **A/tax/ia** is the medical term for not having coordination or order in one's movements. **A/tax/o/phobia** is an abnormal fear of disorder or untidiness. **A/tax/ia/phasia** or **a/tax/a/phasia** is the inability to arrange words into sentences. In surgery, **taxis** means the manual replacement of or reduction of a hernia or dislocation. The surgeon is simply arranging things, putting them in proper order. Taxidermy is the process of arranging the skins (**derm/o**) of animals to look lifelike. In biology, this word part can also refer to the response of an organism to its environment: turning toward a particular stimulus is a positive **taxis;** turning away would be a negative taxis.

From the Latin, **vers/o** means turn. **Vertigo** is dizziness. **Vertiginous** is an adjective that literally means to pertain to **vertigo** but is used more specifically to mean the cause of it. As for non-medical words, there is "version." What is your version of the story? Your spin on the events? And "advertisement," which is meant to turn you towards (the prefix **ad-**) a particular product or service. An aversion for lutefisk? The word tells us that you do not turn towards this delicacy (the prefix **a-** or **an-** means no, not, without).

I hope you've enjoyed learning some new words. There are more in the next chapter!

# Chapter Four

## The Circulatory Systems: Cardiovascular, Blood, and Lymph

*"If you kill a living animal by severing its great arteries, you will find that the veins become empty at the same time as the arteries. This could never happen unless there were anastomoses between them."*
—Galen (*c.* 129–c. 200/216 CE)

### Introduction

In this chapter, we meet the key words of the cardiovascular, the blood, and the lymph systems. The heart is the pumping mechanism of the body; the vascular system has been called the transportation or distribution system of the body. The components of the cardiovascular system are the heart, the blood vessels, and blood. The lymphatic system is sometimes referred to as the drainage system of the body. The component parts are the lymph vessels and the lymph fluid, the lymph nodes and the spleen, thymus, and tonsils.

## Function

Now, we get to the heart of the matter: the heart pumps. That's what it does. No time off. The heart is our hardest-working muscle. We call each contraction a beat and hope our beat is strong and regular. No syncopation here! That's for a jazz band. Each heartbeat pumps blood throughout the body. The blood, traveling through the arteries, veins, and capillaries, carries oxygen, hormones, enzymes, and essential nutrients as well as waste materials. From the minute blood vessels—the capillaries—to the arterioles and venules, then to the arteries and veins, a complete, efficient system exists to get the goods as close as possible to where they are needed: in the cells. The blood flowing through this transportation system is composed of plasma (the fluid), the red blood cells (RBCs), the white blood cells (WBCs), and the platelets.

The function of the lymphatic system is all about immunity and the removal of toxins, waste, and other unwanted materials from the body.

## Key Vocabulary
### Heart

The word **heart** originates in Old English: *heorte.* The number of uses we have for this word indicates its importance to us: from the adjectives "hearty" and "heartless," to "learning something by heart" (to memorize), to "heartburn" (digestion), to "heartland" (geography), to that heartthrob who sometimes causes heartache and even heartbreak. A charming word which comes to us from the Irish *mo chuisle* is "macushla." It is a form of address, as in darling, which literally means my pulse or my heartbeat. How's that for intimacy!

There are two combining forms meaning heart: **card/o** or **cardi/o** and **coron/o**.

1. **Card/o** or **cardi/o** comes to us from the Greek. Examples:
  **cardi/o/megaly**   Because the suffix **-megaly** means large (see the word "mega" in there?), this term refers to an enlarged heart.
  **cardi/o/my/o/pathy**   The suffix **-pathy** comes from the Greek *pathos*. "Pathos" is a word in English as well. It brings to mind poignancy, sympathetic pity, compassion. In the medical world it has evolved into a term meaning disease. The relationship between *pathos* and -pathy could well serve  as  a  reminder to health care practitioners to develop an attitude conducive to a healing environment. The definition of this example is: a disease affecting cardiac muscles.
  **cardi/o/my/o/pexy**    This suffix, **-pexy**, means to fixate, to surgically attach, to put in place. In this case, the surgical fixation or attachment involves cardiac muscle. FYI, a similar suffix is **–desis,** which means fixation or binding.
  **Peri/cardi/um**    The structure (**-um**), membrane surrounding (**peri-**) the heart and the bases of the great vessels. The Greek *peri* means around and is found in "perimeter" (to measure around) and "peripheral" (the line around a circular body; the original meaning referred to the circumference of the earth).

2. **Coron/o,** from the Latin *corona,* means crown or wreath. The **coron/ary arteries** were seen as encircling the upper

heart region and thus crowning the heart. Their purpose is to nourish the heart itself, keeping those coronary muscles pumping. It could be said that the coronary arteries are **coron/oid**, shaped like or resembling a crown.

### Vessels

There are two combining forms referring to the vessels.

1. **Vascul/o** is of Latin derivation: *vasculum* refers to a small vessel. In this chapter, vascul/o is a general term referring to blood and lymph vessels. Examples:
> If an area of the body is richly supplied with blood, it is highly **vascul/ar.**
> I once had a skin tag (an **acro/chordon,** if you want to get technical) that was **a/vascul/ar** (no vessels) and was simply and easily removed by my physician.

2. **Angi/o** is another term referring to blood or lymph vessels and comes from the Greek. Examples:
> **angi/o/plasty**   A procedure involving surgical repair to vessels.
> **angi/o/cardi/o/pathy**   A disease involving the blood vessels of the heart.

### Specific Vessels

**Arter/o** or **arteri/o** derives from the Greek *arteria* meaning—no, not artery or anything to do with blood vessels. The Greek means windpipe. Surprised? There were those among our ancients who, observing that these structures were empty after death, hypothesized that they were air ducts. In medieval times, they were considered to be channels for the vital spirits, vital air, or *pneuma*, which vacated the body at the time of death. Another hypothesis is that an arterial cut allowed vital air to escape and blood to rush in to replace it. The word **trachea** (which we will meet in the chapter on the respiratory system) literally means a rough artery and is so called because of its rings of cartilage.

There are two combining forms referring to the **veins**.

1. **Ven/o** comes from the Latin *vena.* Examples:
   **veni/puncture**   The puncture of a vein, as when one obtains a sample of blood.
   **ven/ectomy**   The surgical removal or resection of a vein.
   **ven/o/clysis**   The suffix is from the Greek *klysis,* which means a washing. The term refers to a continual injection of medicinal or nutritional fluid **intra/ven/ously**.

2. **Phleb/o** means vein as well. The Greek *phlebos* is the source. Examples:
   **phleb/itis**   An inflammation of a vein, most commonly a superficial vein.
   **phleb/o/tom/ist**   A specialist in the opening of veins— well, that's the literal translation. Phlebotomists often work in labs and take blood samples. The word root **tom/o** means to cut.

### Smaller Vessels

**Arteri/ole**   A diminutive of **artery** (**arter/o** or **arteri/o**).

**Ven/ule**   The diminutive of **vein** (**ven/o**).

**Capill/ary** From the Latin *capillaris*, which refers to hair (**pil/i**), perhaps because of the small size or lumen of this vessel.

## Blood

**Hem/o** or **hemat/o** is the combining form which means blood. Examples:

**Hemo/stasis** The stopping of a flow of blood, is assisted in a medical setting such as surgery by use of a **hemo/stat**, an instrument that clamps off a blood vessel, interrupting the flow.

**Hemo/rrhage** A commonly known word. The suffix **-rrhage** means a bursting forth, a profuse flow. In this instance, it is a flowing of blood.

**Hemat/o/logy** The study of blood.

**Hemat/o/chezia** Blood in the stool/feces/bowel movement.

**Hemat/o/poiesis** The process by which blood or blood cells are formed; the suffix **-poiesis** means formation.

**hemo/phil/iac** One who has a tendency to bleed even from minor injuries because their blood's ability to clot is greatly reduced. The suffix **-phil** means to like or love, as in Philadelphia, the city of brotherly love, or "philanthropist," where **anthro** means humankind, but **phil** also refers to a tendency toward, as in **hem/o/phil/ia** (a tendency toward bleeding). And just because you always wanted to know: a nemophilist loves woods or forests, and to be cryophilic is to actually enjoy breaking the ice for a refreshing winter swim. The word means to thrive at low temperatures.

## Additional Vocabulary

**Aort/o** is the combining form for **aorta**. The aorta is the major artery that leaves the heart and divides into branch arteries, and then arterioles, capillaries, venules, and veins. It goes back to the heart via the **venae cavae**, superior and inferior, which form the largest vein in the body.

**Atria** is the plural of **atrium,** and there are two **atria** in the heart. Of the four chambers of the heart, the atria are the two above while the ventricles are below. An atrium is also an open area, open to light. In Roman times, the atrium was the center, the heart, of the home. Sometimes we see atria in hotels or other public places.

**Septum** is a wall or partition, in this case, between the chambers of the heart. There are other **septa** in the body, such as the septum in the nose, which separates the channels or **nares**. Another term meaning a wall or partition is **parietal**. And there is the suffix -**phragm** as in **diaphragm**, which also means a wall or partition.

---

There are **valves** between the four chambers of the heart: the **aortic**, the **pulmonary**, the **tricuspid,** and the **mitral**. Perhaps you noticed the **tri** (three) in tricuspid? **Cusp** means point, so the term means three-pointed.

The word **mitral** comes from the Latin meaning turban; however, the headdress associated with this valve is the mitre worn by Roman Catholic bishops and some abbots. An early anatomist was reminded of the shape of the mitre when studying the heart. This valve is also called the

**bicuspid** and gives us a mnemonic to remember the flow of blood through the heart: Try (tri-) before you buy (bi-).

---

**Ventricle** comes from the Latin and means little belly. This term was first applied to the stomach and then to small cavities in general. A related word is "ventriloquist," which breaks down into **ventri,** meaning belly, and **loqu,** meaning speak. (Someone who is very talkative is described as loquacious.) Ventriloquism means to speak from the belly. A ventriloquist is someone who makes sounds that seem to come from any place but the vocal cords.

The heart pumps and the blood flows. The pumping action creates a **pulse,** a throbbing pressure against the walls of the arteries. One can measure one's pulse wherever the artery is close to the skin. A common point is called the **radial** pulse, because it is the pressure of the fingers on the artery against the **radius** (a bone in the lower arm) that allows one to feel the pulse. Another common pulse point is the **carotid** artery in the neck. Or one can always just go to the source, getting an **apical pulse** by putting the hand or fingers on the chest over the apex of the heart.

Let's pause here to look at the word **apex,** which in adjectival form is **apical**. I remember students challenging me when I would speak of the apex of the heart or the lung and point to a lower portion of the structure. Yes, the word often means the top or highest point of something. The apex of a mountain, the apex of a career, the apex of a certain experience or of a musical work. But in the medical world, it means a narrowed or pointed end of a body part.

The tip of the tongue is the apex of the tongue. The apex of a tooth is the root.

---

Now, to the **blood pressure (BP),** the measurement of the pressure while the heart is contracted compared to when it is at rest. There are two numbers in a blood pressure: 120/80. The upper number is called the **systole** or the **systolic pressure**. The word comes from the Greek meaning a drawing together or a contraction. This number is higher because the heart is pumping and contracting, and the blood is under pressure. The lower number, the **diastole** or **diastolic reading,** is the number reflecting the heart at rest. The Greek source word means dilation. Relaxed, letting it hang out, ready for the next contraction.

The instrument used to determine one's blood pressure is a **sphygm/o/mano/meter. Sphygm/o** means pulse. **Mano** comes from the Greek *manos,* which means thin, rare, loose in texture, porous, scanty, few—in short, occurring at intervals. **Meter** refers to measurement. One needs a **steth/o/scope** to go with the sphygmmm ... the whatchamacallit ... the blood pressure cuff! **Steth/o** originates in the Greek *stethos,* meaning chest, while **-scope** means to view or examine (as in a **bronch/o/scope**) or to observe for a purpose. One does not view anything through a stethoscope—as one can through the variety of scopes used in physical examinations—so in this case the latter definition is the appropriate one: to observe for a purpose. Stethoscopes were first called batons or cylinders. An image search on a computer will show you why.

---

**Plasma** and **serum** are not interchangeable; they are not synonyms. **Serum** is plasma but with the fibrinogen removed or inactivated. With the fibrinogen removed, serum can be handled and tested without it clotting. The term is also sometimes used to mean antiserum or antitoxin. The word comes from the Latin meaning whey (curdling milk). As in "Little Miss Muffett sat on a tuffet eating her curds and whey..." That tuffet may have been a tuft (a grass tuffet) or a footstool or low seat. Since a spider sat down beside her ... but I wander off topic.

**-Stasis** is a suffix meaning to stand or stay in place, to stop. I referred to it above in the words hemo**stat** and hemo**stasis**. Other frequently seen words are **meta/ stasis,** with **meta** referring to beyond or change, as when cancer metastasizes and goes beyond standing still; or **home/o/stasis** where a status quo is the goal. **Home/o** means constant, unchanging, as in homogenized milk; or there is **orthostasis,** standing up straight.

### Maladies and Unwellnesses

**An/echo/ic** means pertaining to being free from echoes or reverberations. Rooms in which certain scientific experiments are conducted need to be **anechoic**.

**An/emia** is a condition marked by a deficiency of red blood cells (which would be **erythr/o/cyt/o/penia**) or of hemoglobin in the blood. There are a variety of types of anemia.

**Aneurysm** is the name for a weakening in an artery wall, or a ballooning out of the vessel wall. The Greek root means dilation. The danger lies in one of these weakened walls bursting. I had a cousin to whom this happened. We were both around twenty-two or twenty-three years old. My cousin had a small daughter, and one day she took her to visit her mother, my aunt. At some point, my cousin complained of a dreadful headache. My aunt suggested that she take aspirin and go lie down for a bit, and she would watch the little one. Those were the last words they exchanged, because my cousin dropped dead from a ruptured aneurysm. It was located in a common place for this ticking time bomb: the base of the brain. Another common aneurysm is known as the "triple A," the **abdominal aortic aneurysm,** which occurs in the lower aorta, in the abdomen.

**Angina pectoris** is often known as **angina** or simply as chest pain. Our ancient predecessors believed that this was a disorder of the chest, not necessarily involving the heart. **Angina** comes from the Latin *angere,* which means to throttle, and the Greek meaning to strangle, while **pectoris** or **pectus** refers to the chest.

**Angi/o/plasty** is a corrective procedure; the suffix **-plasty** means surgical repair, in this case, to a blood vessel.

An **anti/coagulant** slows coagulation, the time it takes for blood to clot. **Anti-** is a prefix meaning against, as in anti-war, anti-globalization, **anti/toxins**, **anti/biotics**.

An **a/rrhythmia,** or a **dys/rhythmia,** is an abnormal cardiac rhythm.

**Ather/o** means fatty plaque. If I told you that **ather/o** comes from a Greek root meaning porridge and that **scler/osis**

is a condition of hardening, you might get a visual image of porridge plastered to the inner walls of your arteries—which would give you an idea of what happens when you eat too much fatty food.

**Brady-** and **tachy-** are two prefixes which, when attached to **cardi/o**, describe opposite characteristics. **Brady/card/ia** is a slow heart rate, and **tachy/card/ia** is a rapid rate.

**Cardi/o/my/o/pathy** is a catch-all term for diseases of the heart muscle. **My/o** means muscle (remember the little mouse?), and the suffix **-pathy** means disease.

**Cardi/o/vascul/ar accident (CVA)** is commonly called a stroke; a historical term that you might still hear is apoplexy.

**Claudication** is a condition that manifests when there is inadequate blood supply to a limb, often the lower leg. It is marked by pain or discomfort and is particularly noticeable when one has been walking or exercising. The Latin verb *claudicare* means to limp, and *claudus* means gait-impaired.

**Cyan/osis** is, literally, a condition of blueness. The skin takes on this bluish quality when there is inadequate oxygenation of the cells. Perhaps you have seen someone who is "blue around the lips."

---

**Echo/cardi/o/gram** is a diagnostic test which uses sound waves to take a moving picture of the heart. This is the second time in this section that I have referred to **echo**. In Greek mythology, there was a mountain nymph named

Echo. She loved the sound of her own voice. She sang and told stories until tragedy struck. As to how this happened, reports vary, but the result was the same: she remains to this day echoing through hill and dale, only able to repeat what someone else has spoken.

**ECG and EKG** Both are abbreviations for an electrocardiogram. **EKG** harks back to the Greek *kardia*, meaning heart.

---

What is the difference between an **embolism** and a **thrombus?** Both are blood clots or other blocking substances. An **embolus** is potentially more dangerous, because it travels, circulating around the body. A **thrombus** is attached to the interior wall of a vessel.

**Fibrillation** is the term for the condition that occurs when the heart muscles are not acting in a coordinated fashion; instead, each is sort of doing its own thing. **Defibrillation** is the stoppage of this erratic activity by means of a **defibrillator,** which administers controlled electrical shocks.

**Ischemia** is the condition of an inadequate blood supply and is particularly used in conjunction with the heart muscles. If **ischemia** lasts too long, it leads to **necr/o/sis**, death of the tissues.

A **my/o/cardi/al infarction** is the medical term for a heart attack. An **infarction** is tissue death (**necrosis**). Don't confuse an infarction with an **infraction,** which is an incomplete bone fracture.

**Palpation** and **palpitation** can easily be confused, too. To **palpate** is to examine by touch, as in: The midwife palpated the pregnant woman's abdomen to determine the position of the fetus. **Palpitation** is a pounding or racing of the heart, uncomfortable sensations in the chest associated with different types of arrhythmias.

**Septic/emia** is a toxicity of the blood. **Sepsis** means infection or toxic and comes from the Greek meaning putrefaction or rot. The suffix **-emia** pertains to the blood.

Anything such as plaque that narrows the vessels causes **stenosis**, which means a condition of narrowing.

A **varicosity** or **varix** (plural **varicies**) is a dilated vein. So, really, to say a varicose vein is redundant, but one hears it all the time.

### The Lymphatic System
### Key Vocabulary

The word **lymph** is from the Latin *lympha,* meaning clear spring water.

The combining form **aden/o** means gland, but when referencing the lymphatic system, it also means **node**. **Lymph/aden/itis** is an inflammation of lymph nodes. By the way, node comes from the Latin *nodus,* meaning 'knob'.

The **thymus** plays a vital role in the effective workings of the body's immune system. Its combining form is **thym/o;** an example would be **thym/o/kinet/ic,** pertaining to the stimulation of the thymus gland.

The **tonsils** are masses of **lymph/oid** tissue (**lymph/oid** literally means resembling **lymphatic** tissue; the tonsils are composed of **lymph/o/cytes**). A spelling note: The word "tonsil" is singular; the word is spelled with one l. The plural is **tonsils**—still one l. Now, when we add the suffixes indicating a medical condition or a treatment, there are two l's as in **tonsill/itis** and **tonsill/ectomy**.

## Additional Vocabulary

The word **immune** comes to us from the Latin *immunis,* which means exempt from public service, or free from taxes. This definition evolved into a medical meaning: to be exempt from a disease. There are two ways to be or become exempt or immune. **Natural immunity** occurs because of a genetic predisposition and is an innate response. This response involves an impressive array of cells ready to defend us. To mention just a few: we have **phag/o/cytes,** where **phag/o** means "to eat," and **macro/ phages,** the humongous eaters of the invading enemy army. Then there are the natural killer cells, known as "NK" in the business. Who says this isn't exciting?

**Acquired immunity** is of two types: active (because of having a disease, or getting a vaccination, or receiving a transfer of immune cells from a donor) and passive (because of having antitoxins, immunoglobulins, or maternal antibodies—through mother's milk, for example). The immunoglobulins are antibodies present in the body's fluids or **humors.** Did you know that research has shown that feelings of guilt may damage the immune system by lowering the immunoglobulin levels? Forgiveness of oneself and others is good for your health!

---

Now, the term **humor** dates all the way back to Hippocrates (c. 460 – c. 377 BCE) and his theory of body humors.

Hippocrates strongly held to a rule of harmony. All body systems were to be in balance, and disease resulted from imbalance. He taught the importance of balance between the four bodily fluids, or humors (also spelled "humours"): blood, phlegm, yellow bile, and black bile. Each **humor** (the Latin word for fluid) was associated with a specific personality characteristic.

1.  Blood (*sanguis*) is the sanguine personality: sturdy, confident, optimistic, passionate and cheerful. To be consanguineous is to have a familial relationship with someone, to be of the same blood.
2.  Phlegm (*phlegma*) is the phlegmatic personality: stolid, cool, impassive, sluggish, dull.
3.  Choler (from *khole*, referring to yellow bile) is a quality or state of being irascible. To be choleric is to be irritable, quick tempered without apparent cause. **Cholera** means yellow as in yellow fever. "Bilious" (from *bilis*, also yellow bile) was used to describe a person who was peevish or ill natured. "To have gall" was to be bitter, insolent, or rancorous. This would describe someone acting with an imbalance of spleen mingling ill will with bad temper. And "to be jaundiced" was to be envious or hostile.
4.  Black bile (*melancholia*) is the melancholic personality. Coming from the Greek for sadness, it was to be depressed, sad. *Melan* means black.

The physician's task was to help restore balance or harmony. Treatments used towards that end included emetics, cathartics, purgatives, and bloodletting.

Another treatment was the use of hot plasters. Sophia Peabody Hawthorne, wife of American author Nathaniel Hawthorne, suffered from severe migraines. She blistered her skin with hot plasters to draw off pernicious internal humors in an effort to remedy her headaches.

Bloodletting was used to reduce excess circulation, to slow the pulse, and to minimize irritation, all felt to be the cause of inflammation.

I find it interesting to note how many of these terms are still in use today. Granted, some are not in common usage, but we still refer to someone being ill-humored, or melancholic, or phlegmatic, or sanguine.

Ayruvedic medicine, an ancient medical system from India, also has a theory of bodily humors, as do the Chinese and indigenous Americans.

### Maladies and Unwellnesses

**AIDS,** the acronym for **acquired immunodeficiency syndrome,** is a late stage in the infection caused by the **human immunodeficiency virus (HIV).**

An **auto/immune disorder,** we know from the prefix **auto-,** has something to do with one's own self as opposed to an external source. Indeed, this is a disease produced when the body's normal tolerance of the antigens on its own cells is disrupted. An **opportunistic infection** is one that attacks the body when the immune system is already compromised, taking advantage of the situation, so to speak.

**Aller/gen** is the name given to any substance that causes a hypersensitivity reaction or abnormal immune response. **Ana/phylaxis** is an exaggerated allergic response, rapid in onset and potentially life-threatening, found in individuals who have had a previous encounter with the guilty allergen.

**Anti/biotics** literally means against life, in this case the life of microorganisms. It refers to any substance that destroys or inhibits the growth of those ever-so-tiny creatures.

An **anti/gen** (literally, against producing) is a substance that initiates or causes the production of an **anti/body.** Why does it do that? Because the antigen is a foreign or toxic substance that enters the body, triggering the antibody unique to that antigen and rendering the antigen ineffective. A superhero molecule uniquely formed for the occasion.

**Bacteria** is the plural for **bacterium,** the proper term for one of these single-cell organisms. Some are bad and are called **pathogens** (literally, disease producing), but many are very **beneficial,** which comes from the Latin *bene* (well) and *facere* (make).

**Carcin/oma (in situ)** is a **mal/ign/ant** tumor originating in body tissue. **Mal-** means bad. Think malware, maladjusted, maltreated, malice, malign, malediction (the opposite of benediction), and so on. A malignancy is prone to spread, which is called **meta/stasis. Stasis** means standing, remember, while **meta** is beyond, so the tumor or mass

(**-oma**) has gone beyond standing still. **In situ** indicates a static situation. This Latin phrase refers to something that is in its original place or position, and our word "situate" is a derivative. *In situ* indicates an early stage in the development of the carcinoma, before metastasis has occurred.

In **hemo/lysis,** the suffix **-lysis** means to break down, dissolve, loosen, separate. The word **hemo/lytic** refers to the destruction of red blood cells: **hem/o** means blood. An **anxi/o/lytic** is something that reduces anxiety, breaking it down and dissolving it; the term is usually used in reference to a drug. As well, there is "analysis" and Lysol.

A **macro/phage** or a **macro/phag/o/cyte** is a big eater. Literally. **Macro** means large as in "mega," and **phage** comes from the Greek meaning to eat. It's what these cells eat that earns them my thanks; they assist in the destruction of those antigens, bacteria, and viruses, for example.

**Splen/o/megaly** refers to an enlarged spleen. The suffix is a form of **mega** again: **megaly**.

**Toxins:** The ancient Greeks (among others) smeared poison on arrowheads used in hunting. The Greek *toxikon* translates as "arrow poison," and the Greek word *toxon* refers to a bow, so these words had to do with archery. A toxophilite is a lover of archery. Interestingly, the Greek *pharmakon* can be translated as "cure" and "poison." One might say, the poison applied to that arrow. Today, the combining form **toxic/o** or **tox/o** has come to mean poison. A **toxicologist** is one who specializes in the study of poisons, while a **pharmacist** is a specialist in the dispensing of medicines/drugs.

**Vaccination** comes from the Latin word for cow. In Spanish, the word is similar: *vaca*. (In Tucson, Arizona, there is a street named Camino Sin Vacas, or Road Without Cows! I love it!). Edward Jenner (1749-1823), an English physician and scientist, observed that cow maids didn't get the disfiguring and often fatal smallpox that was so common in that time. They got the much milder disease of cowpox. He theorized that the acquired immunity to cowpox gave them immunity to smallpox as well. He was so sure that injecting a person with cowpox organisms would protect them from the dreaded smallpox that the first person he tested his theory on was his son. The resultant process of introducing altered antigens to produce an immune response and protection against disease he called "vaccination."

**Varicella** is the medical term for chickenpox, which is caused by the varicella zoster virus. Chickenpox is a common childhood disease, but this virus has a nasty ability to remain dormant (sleeping) until later in life when it bursts out as **herpes zoster**, also known as **shingles**.

So many words! So little time! On to the next chapter...

# Chapter Five
## The Endocrine System

*"Your medicine is in you, and you do not observe it. Your ailment is from yourself and you do not register it."*
—Hazrat Ali, Sufi master (600–61 CE)

### Introduction

The endocrine system is a communication system. This system, along with the nervous system, regulates the various functions or processes of the body. The endocrine system does this through glands, which secrete hormones that are in turn disbursed through the bloodstream. The nervous system uses neurotransmitters and electrical impulses to communicate. The primary link between these two systems is the **hypothalamus,** which is located in the lower central part of the brain.

### Function

The purpose of the endocrine system is to keep the body in homeostasis or equilibrium so that all body systems can function optimally, at their best. It does this through the production and regulation of hormones in glands.

# Key Vocabulary
## Hormones

**Hormone** comes from the Greek meaning to set in motion, to urge on, excite. The hormones can be powerful instigators of action! These extremely potent chemicals have been compared to changing the color of Lake Michigan from blue to red just by dropping a few drops of red food coloring into the lake! In years past, I have observed workers in small boats dumping buckets of green dye into the Chicago River, changing it to an Irish green for St. Patrick's Day. Compare that to adding a few drops to Lake Michigan! Wow. After considering this, a female student in one of my classes exclaimed, "No wonder women have mood swings or PMS (pre-menstrual syndrome)!" Another student commented on the difficulty of managing HRT (hormone replacement therapy). And now, recall those hormone surges of puberty...

Each hormone affects only its target cells, the ones that have receptors for that specific hormone. They then alter the metabolism of that target cell.

## Glands

**Glands** are the source, the secretors of the hormones in the endocrine system. The combining form for gland is **aden/o.** Examples:

> **aden/ec/top/ia**   The condition of a gland being out of (**ec-** means out of or outside) place (**top/o** means

place, position, location), or not in its normal position.
**aden/oid**   An object resembling (**-oid**) a gland.
**aden/o/gen/ous**  Pertaining to originating in glandular tissue.
**aden/o/cellul/itis**   Inflammation of a gland and the cellular tissue adjacent to it.

**Endo/crine** breaks down into the prefix **endo-,** which means within, and the word root **crine** (the combining form is **crin/o**), which means to secrete. The **endocrine** glands secrete hormones into the bloodstream, within the body. The bloodstream provides an efficient distribution system that gives access to all cells of the body. Now, the body also has **ex/o/crine glands,** which secrete to the outside of the body. **Ex-** means from, away from, out of. Examples of **exocrine** glands are the sweat, salivary, tear or lacrimal, and mammary glands.

## Specific Glands

The **pituitary** is known as the **Master Gland** as it secretes hormones that act on other endocrine glands. (It tells other endocrine glands what to do). *Pituita* is the Latin from which this gland takes its name. It translates as slime, phlegm, mucus, catarrh. The ancients thought that nasal mucus was channeled from the pituitary gland. The pituitary is located in the **sella turcica** of the sphenoid bone in the brain. *Sella turcica* is Latin for Turkish saddle. The Greek **hypo/phy/sis** refers to the location of the pituitary gland. Starting with the suffix, the word means the condition (**-sis**) of growing (**phys**) under or below (**hypo**).

Other glands in the endocrine system include: the **pineal**, **thyroid**, **parathyroid** (four of them), **thymus**, **adrenal** (two of these), **pancreas**, **gonads** (two testes or two ovaries, depending on your gender) plus specialized cells in tissues throughout the body.

The **pineal** is so named because of its shape; the word is from the Latin meaning pine cone.

The **thyroid** means resembling (**-oid**) a shield.

The prefix **para-** means near, beside, alongside of. The **parathyroid glands** are near, beside, the thyroid.

The prefix **ad-** means to or toward, and **renal** means pertaining to the kidney. That's where the **adrenals** are, adjacent to the kidney.

Finally, the **pancreas** comes to us from the Latinized Greek. *Pan* means all, entire, and *kreas* means flesh. You will also find it translated as sweetbread, a culinary delicacy for some.

We'll meet the thymus when discussing the lymph system and the gonads in the chapter on the reproductive system.

## Additional Vocabulary

**Andr/o/gen** is the male sex hormone. **Andro** means male and **-gen** means to produce.

**Ant/agon/ism** is the process in which two hormones exert opposite effects on their target cells, while **syn/erg/**

**ism** is the process where two hormones work together to get a result.

A **cortex** and **medulla** are found in various parts of the body. In this chapter, I am spotlighting the **adren/al gland**. This gland has an outer portion, or layer, called the **cortex;** in the Latin, the word cortex refers to the bark of a tree, an outer covering. The **medulla** refers to the middle or median; the word means marrow or pith.

**Endo/crin/o/logy** is the field of study concentrating on hormones and **endo/crine** glands and their accompanying disorders.

**Estro/gen** takes us back to our Greek forebears. This is the female sex hormone, and it takes its name from *oistros*, which is Greek for gadfly. It also means the insect's sting. Now, a stinging insect can excite to action, even madness, frenzy. And from there the word came to be used in conjunction with the reproductive cycle in women. There is more: a story involving a young girl named Io, who was desired by Zeus (was there ever a young girl not desired by Zeus?), a jealous wife named Hera, a heifer, a peacock, and a stinging gadfly. I'll let you look that one up at your leisure.

**Eu/thyr/oid/ism** is the condition (**-ism**) of having a normally functioning (**eu-**) thyroid gland.

**Fasting blood sugar** is a diagnostic test to determine how much glucose (sugar) is in a blood sample after an overnight fast. The **hemoglobin A1c** test, or simply the A1c test, indicates one's average blood sugar level for the past two to three months.

**Inhibition,** in this context, is the action of a hormone to prevent an endocrine gland from secreting its hormones.

**Islets of Langerhans** are found in the pancreas. This is where insulin is produced.

**Melatonin** is a hormone secreted by the pineal gland. It helps control the sleep/wake (**circadian**) cycles. Don't confuse this with melanin, which is a dark brown or black pigment—remember, *melas* is Greek for black.

### Maladies and Unwellnesses

Dysfunctions in hormone production are either a deficiency, a **hypo/secretion**, or an excess, a **hyper/secretion**.

In **acr/o/megaly**, the suffix **-megaly** means enlargement, and the combining form **acr/o** refers to extremities or top. These clues lead us toward a condition in which the pituitary gland produces an excessive amount of growth hormone in an adult person. It is chronic and results in abnormal growth of the hands, feet, and face.

The term **ad/ren/o/cortic/o/hyper/plasia** is a reminder that long words can be easily understood when broken down into their component parts. Starting with the suffix **-plasia**—which has to do with development, formation, growth—we note that this is **hyper** or excessive growth involving the **adrenal cortex**.

In **calci/penia**, the suffix **-penia** means deficiency, in this case a deficiency of calcium. The term **hypo/calc/emia** is more specific in that it indicates the shortage is in the blood.

**Cretinism** is a **con/genit/al** (pertaining to being present at birth) condition. There is a lack of thyroid hormones which, if left untreated, results in severely stunted physical growth and mental retardation.

**Cushing's Syndrome** is caused by a **hypersecretion** of the adrenal cortex.

---

**Diabetes insipidus** and **mellitus**: Have you ever known anyone with an insipid personality—dull and flat? That is a clue to the name of a less common form of diabetes, **insipidus**, which, because of frequent urination, is characterized by diluted urine. **Diabetes insipidus** is caused by a **hyposecretion** of a pituitary hormone or a failure of the kidney to respond to this hormone.

By contrast, the more common **mellitus** (as in **diabetes mellitus**) means honey, sweet. The term **glucose** comes from the Greek meaning sweet. Back in the day before sophisticated laboratories, taste-testing detected the sweetness present in certain urine samples (caused by excessive amounts of glucose) and the blandness or insipidness of others. This observation was combined with the presence of such symptoms as **poly/ur/ia** (**poly** means many, and **ur/ia** refers to urine) or frequent urination, and **poly/dips/ia** (the combining form **dips/o** means thirst) or frequent thirst. This assisted in the determination of a diagnosis. Another term starting with **poly-** is among the symptoms of diabetes mellitus: **poly/phagia** or excessive hunger and eating. By the way, polyuria can also be caused by an excessive intake of fluids—especially coffee!—or by diuretic medications.

---

**Graves disease** is a condition caused by **hyper/thyr/oid/ ism**. It was first described by Dr. Robert Graves (1796-1853), an English physician and pathologist. There are a variety of possible signs and symptoms with Graves. Two might need a bit of explanation. The first is **goiter,** which comes from the Latin *guttur,* meaning throat, and is caused by an iodine deficiency. The second is **ex/ophthalmos,** which literally means out, from, away from the eye. The bulging, protruding eye exposes most of the white of the eye, giving an individual a staring or startled expression.

When women grow hair on their body in places where men usually have hair, it is called **hirsutism**. There can be a variety of causes, and one of them is endocrine-related: the excessive production of **andr/o/gens** from the **ad/ren/ al** glands.

**Hirsutism** and several other terms in this chapter end in the suffix **–ism,** which means process or condition. It has several other meanings as well. In plagiarism, for example, it means an act, practice, or process. It means a distinctive practice, system, or philosophy when used in Buddhism, Confucianism, liberalism, etc.

**Hyper/kal/emia** or **hypo/kal/emia** refers to the condition of excessive or deficient potassium **(kal/i)** in the blood.

**Myxedema** is a severe or advanced form of **hypo/thyr/oid/ism**.

Keep up the good work!

# Chapter Six
## The Nervous System

*"Pronoia (as opposed to paranoia) is the sneaking suspicion that the whole world is conspiring to shower you with blessings. Symptoms include sudden attacks of optimism and outbreaks of goodwill."*
—Anonymous

### Introduction

Your body's nervous system is a very complex piece of work. It is comprised of the brain and the spinal cord, which together make up the control center or central nervous system, as well as that vast network of nerves throughout the whole body that constitutes the peripheral nervous system.

### Function

The nervous system monitors changes in the environment inside and outside the body; this information is provided by the sense organs. The nervous system interprets the changes, initiates the response, and, with the endocrine system, works to maintain homeostasis.

# Key Vocabulary
## Brain

The **brain** has two combining forms: **cerebr/o** and **encephal/o**.

1. **Cerebr/o** is used to refer to the **brain** as a whole as well as referring to the **cerebr/um**, which is the largest part of the brain. The Latin word *cerebrum* means brain. Examples:

**cerebr/al**  Pertaining to the brain; the term can refer to a person who "lives in his/her head" and is more in touch with their intellect than their emotions or intuition. As a medical term, this word is frequently seen as an adjective that modifies nouns that specify a condition, such as:

• **cerebr/al aneurysm**  A weakened blood vessel in the brain which balloons and sometimes bursts.

• **cerebr/al thromb/osis**  A condition of having a clot that is stationary.

• **cerebr/al embol/ism**  Indicates a blockage, generally a blood clot in the brain that has traveled through the vascular system.

• **cerebr/al palsy**  A condition of partial paralysis usually caused by brain damage before or at birth.

2. **Encephal/o** literally translates to in (**en-**) the head (**cephal**). What is in the head? The brain. This combining form comes from the Greek.  Examples:

**encephal/itis**  Inflammation of the brain.

**an/encephal/y**  A congenital condition in which all or a major part of the brain is missing.

**encephal/o/graphy**   The process of recording the structure and electrical activity of the brain.

## Spinal Cord

**Myel/o** is the combining form for both the spinal cord and bone marrow. References to bone marrow are in the musculoskeletal chapter while an example referring to the spinal cord is given below. Example:

> **myel/auxe**   .An abnormal enlargement of the spinal cord; the suffix **-auxe** refers to increase.

## Nerves

**Neur/o** is the combining form used when signifying a nerve. A **neur/on** is a nerve cell which is the structural and functional unit of the nervous system. Examples:

> **neur/o/pathy**   A catch-all term for diseases involving the nerves.
> **neur/ectasia**   A condition of surgically stretching (**-ectasia**) a nerve.
> **neur/algia**   Pain occurring along the course of a nerve.
> **neur/o/clon/ic**   Pertaining to nervous spasms (**clon**). The noun clonus refers to spasms.

# Additional Vocabulary
## Central and Peripheral Nervous Systems

The **central nervous system (CNS)** consists of the brain and spinal cord.

The **peripheral nervous system (PNS)** consists of all the rest of the nervous system.

One component of the PNS is the set of **cranial nerves**. Many, many years ago, when I was a student nurse, we were taught the following mnemonic to help us remember the names and order of the cranial nerves. More recent students assure me that it is still in use, along with a variety of other mnemonics which may assist in learning this list.

| On | Olfactory |
|---|---|
| Old | Optic |
| Olympus' | Oculomotor |
| Towering | Trochlear |
| Top | Trigeminal |
| A | Abducens |
| Finn | Facial |
| And | Auditory (or vestibulocochlear) |
| German | Glossopharyngeal |
| Viewed | Vagus |
| Some | Spinal |
| Hops | Hypoglossal |

**Afferent nerves** are the sensory nerves; they carry nerve impulses toward the CNS from the sensory organs. The Latin root of **afferent** has to do with bringing to or towards.

**Efferent nerves** are the motor nerves. The Latin source means to bring away from. Here, the nerve impulses are going out from the CNS to the muscles or glands to effect the orders of the body's control center.

**Autonomic** refers to functions that are unconsciously controlled; they are involuntary or reflexive, such as the body's "fight or flight" response. The **autonomic nervous system** is part of the PNS.

**Somatic** refers to the voluntarily controlled movements of the body using the skeletal muscles. The **somatic nervous system** is part of the PNS.

## More Additional Vocabulary

**Alges/o** is a combining form indicating pain. We have already met this word part in its form as a suffix: **-algia**. You can see an example of its use as a combining form in the word **an/alges/ia,** pertaining to being without pain.

In Latin, **cauda equina** translates to tail of a horse. Located at the bottom end of the spinal cord, all those nerve endings emerge resembling, to some, the tail of a horse.

**Cerebrospinal fluid (spinal fluid)** is found circulating within the brain and spinal cord.

**Cognition** comes from the Latin meaning knowledge. It refers to the mental processes of acquiring knowledge, understanding, thinking, and remembering.

**Conscious** comes to us from the Latin meaning to be aware. It's all about awareness, responding to one's environment, being awake. In a spiritual sense, it is used to indicate one who is fully in the moment.

**Esthes/o** is the combining form denoting sensation. Examples:

> **an/esthes/ia**   The condition of being without sensation.
>
> **par/esthes/ia**   The condition of irregular or abnormal sensation; used specifically to denote tingling, prickly

sensations caused by pressure or damage to a peripheral nerve.

**Esthe/tics** indicates an awareness and appreciation for beauty and art. An **esthe/tician** in dentistry is concerned with the appearance of a dental restoration. The **medical esthe/tician** is concerned with skincare, particularly facial skincare. The suffix **-tician** is a combination of the suffix **–tic,** meaning pertaining to, and the suffix **–ician,** which refers to a specialist, someone skilled in a particular area.

**Ganglion** (plural **ganglia**) means swelling or knot. A ganglion occurs where one finds a nerve cell cluster. When connected with other ganglia, a ganglion has a **plexus**, which is the Latin for braid. These connections provide intermediary junctions or relay points on the complex highway of the nerves. (A ganglion can also refer to a benign tumor that has formed on a tendon.)

*Glia* is the Greek word for glue. **Neuro/gli/al cells** support and protect the nerve cells, the neurons.

**Gyrus** (plural **gyri**) and **sulcus** (plural **sulci**) refer to the convoluted hills and valleys in the topography of the brain. The gyri are the elevations, and the sulci are the grooves. In Latin *sulcus* means furrow or ditch.

**Mening/o** is the combining form for the **meninges** (singular **meninx**).The meninges are protective layers or membranes covering the brain and spinal cord. The outermost layer has been named the **dura mater**; next are the **arachnoid membrane** and, innermost, the **pia mater**. The names of the two outer layers come to us from the Latin *mater*, meaning mother, as in "maternity"; *dura* meaning hard or tough as in "durable"; *pia* referring to tenderness. The arachnoid membrane was identified later than the other two and was given the descriptive name "resembling a spider or web." The Greek *arakhne* means spider or spider's web and the suffix **-oid** means resembling. In the **subarachnoid** space flows the **cerebrospinal fluid**.

Neuron parts: When you can, do a computer search for an image of a **neuron**, so that these labels of the main parts of the nerve cell will have greater significance. We start with the **dendrites**, which get their name from the Greek word for tree —good name, right? Next is the **soma** or body of the nerve cell. Then the *axon*, which is the Greek word for axis. The **myelin sheath** (a sheath is a close-fitting cover such as the scabbard of a sword; "scabbard" is another word for sheath or vagina, a condom, or a woman's dress style) acts as an electrical insulator and increases the velocity of nerve impulse transmission. The **terminal end fibers** are also called **axon terminals** or **synaptic knobs**, **terminal** or **end buttons**, or **boutons**. Finally, the **synapse**. The Greek *synapsis* means connection or junction. There is actually a space, albeit very small, between nerve cells. This distance is crossed by **neurotransmitters** such as acetylcholine, dopamine, epinephrine, serotonin, and a whole lot more. The idea of the synapse, the space, has been used as a symbol or metaphor for potential in such fields as transpersonal psychology.

**Neur/o/plasticity** or **brain plasticity** (the suffix **-plasticity** pertains to formation) is the brain's awesome ability to reorganize itself, to form new connections or synapses throughout life. This rewiring may occur after a trauma to the brain or a stroke, or through the influence of experience. Old, unused connections are deleted in a process called **synaptic pruning**. As in "Don't use it, ya' lose it." Repetition, practicing a musical instrument, or telling stories in the tradition of oral historians strengthen the neural connections. Bonus word: Someone who begins to learn or study a new subject area late in life is an "opsimath."

---

Listen up! The following discussion of **psych/o**, **ment/o**, and **phren/o** may prove a bit—okay, more than a bit—confusing, but we will take it one combining form at a time. The English word is "mind." We will consider three combining forms used to indicate the mind. One comes from the Latin (**ment/o** as in **mental** or **dementia**). The other two come to us from Greek origins (**psych/o** as in **psychotherapy** and **phren/o** as in **schizophrenia**). The Greek *psycho* originally meant something closer to soul, the essence of life, but it has evolved into its present usage.

Now, here's the part that can be confusing: **phren/o** means both mind and diaphragm! Depending on whether one is using **phren/o** from the Greek, meaning mind, or **phren/o** from the Latin, meaning diaphragm. **Phren/o/dynia** means a pain in the diaphragm. **Phren/ic** means pertaining to the diaphragm. In this context **phren/o** comes from the Latin derivation. The context in which the word is used determines whether it is the diaphragm or the mind that is under discussion.

A bit of trivia: Have you ever heard of **phrenology**? (And here I am referring to the Greek root meaning mind.) A German physician, Franz Joseph Gall, was among the first to note, in 1796, that different parts of the brain have specific functions. Phrenology became very popular in Victorian times. It analyzed the shapes of the subjects' heads for signs of strength and weakness in mind and character. Throughout the nineteenth century, it was the most widely credited science of the mind. In 1832, it was accepted by the Boston Medical Society and was on the curriculum at Harvard Medical School. The sense that the brain could be studied as a factor in human behavior has proven to be prescient. One can still purchase a **phrenology skull** with its mind map.

---

**Radicul/o** sometimes shortened to **radic/o**, means nerve root and comes from the Latin *radix,* from which we get "radical" or "eradicate." Weeds are eradicated when they are taken out, roots and all. Or, think of this word when eating a radish—a root vegetable. **Radicul/itis**, or inflammation of a nerve root, is also known as a pinched nerve. **Radicul/o/pathy** is the collective term for disease conditions of nerve roots.

The Greek equivalent for the nerve root is **rhiz/o.** For botanists, this calls to mind the rhizome, a type of plant root. **Rhyz/o/tomy** indicates an incision into a nerve root.

### Maladies and Unwellnesses

**Alzheimer's disease** is the most common type of **dementia** in older adults. The word **de/ment/ia** comes from the Latin meaning a condition (**-ia**) of lacking (**de-**) of mind (**ment**) or out of one's mind. Named for the German neuropathologist and psychiatrist, Alois Alzheimer (1864-1915), it is a disorder of the mental processes characterized by memory problems, personality changes, and impaired reasoning.

---

Following is a short listing of **a-** (meaning no, not, without) words which tie in with brain function:

**a/kinet/ic**   Pertaining to the loss or impairment of movement.

**a/mnes/ia**   From the Greek meaning forgetfulness, a loss or impairment of memory.

**a/phas/ia**   The loss or impairment of speech (not to be confused with **a/phagia,** the inability to eat or swallow). The Greek *aphatos* means speechless and is the basis for this term. The next time you are rendered speechless by a surprise or a startling event, you will be temporarily **a/phas/ic**.

**a/prax/ia**   The inability to perform purposive movements; **echo/prax/ia** is the   imitation of an action. Toddlers are good at this! As are teens, within their peer group.

**a/tax/ia**   A lack of full control of one's bodily movements, lacking co-ordination.

---

Back to our regular listing:

**-asthenia** is a suffix that pertains to weakness; an example is **my/asthen/ia gravis**, a serious or grave (**gravis**) condition of muscular (**my**) weakness (**esthenia**).

**Aut/ism** literally translates to a condition (**-ism**) of the self (**aut/o**). In classic psychiatry, it is defined as a mental introversion. I am thinking of a child I knew when I was a staff nurse at a state mental hospital many years ago. He was almost totally within his own world, exhibited repetitive movements such as banging his head against walls, was expert at climbing the interlocking metal link covering on the high windows, and whistled beautifully. Nowadays, **autism** is a spectrum of developmental disorders marked by communication and social issues, focused interests, and repetitive behaviors. **Aut/o** comes from the Greek, while the Latin for self is **sui** as in **sui/cide** (to kill oneself).

**Bipolar disorder** is a condition marked by alternating states of elation and depression; it was formerly known as **manic depression**.

**Caus/o** is the combining form for caustic, burning. **Caus/algia** is a burning pain.

**Cephal/algia** is a headache.

**Cerebrovascular accident (CVA)** is also called a **stroke** or **apoplexy**; there are two types of CVA: **hemorrhagic** and **ischemic**, the latter referring to an obstruction to the flow of blood. A **transient ischemic attack (TIA)**, or mini-stroke, is the temporary interruption in the blood supply to the brain.

**Coma** is the Greek for deep sleep or trance.

**Concuss/o**, as in **concussion,** comes from the Latin meaning to shake together; it is an injury resulting from impact with an object.

**Convuls/o**, as in **convulsion**, comes to us from the Latin and refers to a sudden violent muscular contraction.

**Encephal/itis**, literally an inflammation of the brain, has been known historically as sleeping sickness and is an inflammation of the white and gray matter of the brain.

**Epi/lepsy:** The combining form is **epileps/o** and comes from the Greek meaning to lay hold of or seize (**leps**) upon (**epi-**). Those early Greeks called this "the Sacred Disease" as they interpreted the attacks as one being seized upon by the gods in retribution for some offense. An unknown author writing around 400 BCE is credited with being the first to offer a physiological cause for the seizure. Using the Hippocratic humor theory, the writer described the condition as having to do with the flux of the phlegm—a bodily humor or humour—flowing through the brain rather than divine intervention. Epilepsy has also been called "the falling sickness" or a "fit," and mistletoe or thrush twig has been used to treat it in days past. At one point, putting a paper bag over one's head was thought to provide a cure. There are two primary categories of seizures: the **grand mal**, which I have heard compared to an electrical storm in the brain, and the **petit mal**, which can be as minimal as a flickering eyelid.

**Hallucinate** or **hallucination** comes from a Latin verb which means to wander in the mind; a **hallucination** is a false perception having no relation to reality.

**Herpes Zoster** or **shingles** is a viral infection of the peripheral nerves.

**Huntington's disease** is a **neuro/de/generative** (loss of structure or function, degeneration of neurons) disease. This condition has been called **Huntington's chorea**. *Chorea* comes from both the Greek and the Latin and means dance. This leads to the other historical name for this disease, **St. Vitus Dance**, a reference to the involuntary movements exhibited by a person. When I was a very little girl, a dear family friend had what was then called St. Vitus Dance. Her movements and speech were difficult, but she was able to take care of housekeeping duties for my grandfather after the death of his wife.

**Hydro/cephalus** has been known commonly as "water on the brain"; it is the accumulation of excessive amounts of cerebrospinal fluid within the brain.

---

**Migraine, prodrome,** and **aura:** Welcome to my world. I can't just write that a migraine comes from the Greek meaning **hemi-** (or half) skull. Or that it is a familial disorder marked by periodic, usually unilateral (one-sided) pulsing headaches that begin in childhood or early adult life and tend to recur with diminishing frequency in later life. I was three years old when a child specialist (we would now say a "pediatrician") in the city nearest to our rural home diagnosed me as having migraines. I was the youngest subject he had ever seen, he told my parents. Well, we all must have our claim to fame.

A **prodrome** is a sign or symptom that comes before or precedes the disorder. A rash before a fever is an example. **Pro-** means before, prior, preceding, or in front of; it also means favoring or supporting as in taking a pro-peace stand (so much more positive sounding than anti-war). A **probiotic,** a microorganism introduced into the body for its beneficial qualities, is another example.

An **aura** in this context refers to a sensation sometimes perceived by a person before a migraine attack, or an epileptic seizure, or other conditions involving the brain. When I experience an aura, it is usually a zigzag line in my visual field. Some experience other visual aura or sensory perceptions.

---

**Narc/o/lepsy** translates as being seized by (**-lepsy**) sleep or stupor (**narco**). Narcolepsy points to a deficiency in the neurotransmitter hypocretin and certain brain abnormalities that might affect the regulation of the sleep/wake cycle.

**Paranoia** literally means pertaining to an irregular mind; feelings of persecution, being suspicious, discriminated against.

**Parkinson's disease** is a condition that has also been called Parkinsonism, paralysis agitans, and shaking palsy. In 1817, Dr. James Parkinson, an English physician, wrote "An Essay on the Shaking Palsy." This is a chronic, degenerative disease of the central nervous system.

**Phobia** comes from the Greek *phobos,* meaning terror, panic. It is defined as excessive or irrational fear and is a common suffix or a noun standing on its own. There are so many examples to choose from, but here is my list:

   **acro/phobia**   heights
   **agora/phobia**   open spaces (*agora* is Greek for marketplace)
   **ailuro/phobia**   cats

**andro/phobia**  men
**claustro/phobia**  confined space
**cyno/phobia**  dogs
**gamo/phobia**  marriage
**gyne/phobia**  women
**hemo/phobia**  blood
**ochlo/phobia**  crowds
**phobo/phobia**  fear of developing a phobia
**photo/phobia**  light (This term can also mean a sensitivity to light, which, of course is not an irrational fear.)
**thanato/phobia**  death
**xeno/phobia**  strangers

**Poli/o/myel/itis** is often shortened to **polio**; historically, it was called infantile paralysis. Broken down, the term means inflammation (**-itis**) of the gray (**poli/o**) matter of the spinal cord (**myel**).

**Psych/iatr/y** literally means the process (**-y**) of treating (**iatr**) the mind (**psych**).

**Psycho/sis** is a state of severe emotional disturbance in which there is an impaired relationship with what most people think of as reality. (Who said "Reality is the only word in the English language that should always be used in quotes?" I would add the word "normal" as another such word.) A **delusion** is a firmly held belief that is contradicted by generally accepted reality. Examples are a delusion of grandeur or of persecution.

**Psych/o/somat/ic** pertains to mind (**psych/o**) and body (**somat/o**); the relationship between them. It usually refers to physical disorders with psychological causes.

**Post-traumatic stress disorder (PTSD) is** a mental health condition that's triggered by experiencing or witnessing a terrifying event.

**Somn/o** is the combining form for sleep. Examples:

**somn/ambulate** To walk in one's sleep.

**somni/loquy** A sleep disorder; the act of talking in one's sleep. (In Latin, *loqui* means to speak.) How loquacious are you when asleep?

**in/somn/ia** That frustrating condition (**-ia**) of not (**in-**) sleeping.

**para/somn/ia** Any disorder characterized by abnormal or unusual behavior of the nervous system during sleep.

The prefix **syn-** in **syn/drome** means together. The word root **drome** comes from the Greek *dromos,* which refers to a running or race course. Think of a dromedary, a type of camel which can be raced. The word **syndrome** refers to a grouping of signs or symptoms that occur together (run together). An assignment that I used in classes when I was teaching resulted in quite a fascinating listing of syndromes: shaken baby syndrome, uncontrollable hair syndrome, phantom vibration syndrome, Tourette's syndrome, 1p36 deletion syndrome, Asperger Syndrome, Down Syndrome, restless leg syndrome, fetal alcohol syndrome, toxic shock syndrome, Stockholm syndrome, Munchausen syndrome and Munchausen by proxy, Prader Willi syndrome, post-traumatic stress syndrome, musical ear syndrome, Ekbom syndrome—Euwww... I get a creepy, crawly sensation, just writing that one. A student wrote a passionate email to me about the black dog (or cat) syndrome. Do a search on any or all of these syndromes.

**Syn/cope** is a temporary loss of consciousness caused by a drop in blood pressure; fainting.

**Therapy** and **therapeutic** have to do with the process of curing or healing from disease.

**Tourette syndrome** is a neurological disorder marked by repetitive muscular and verbal tics.

**Tic douloureux**: **Tic** is a French word meaning a habitual spasmodic contraction, while **douloureux** means painful. This condition is also known as **tri/gemin/al neur/algia.**

You were warned! There is much that is complex about the nervous system. But isn't it fascinating as well? I hope you want to delve deeper and learn more.

# Chapter Seven
## The Senses

### Introduction

The senses are all about perception. To perceive is to receive and collect information through the capacity of the five senses (and don't forget the sixth sense, intuition) to provide the brain with information about the external environment and assist us in understanding and responding to the world around us. We will give most attention in this chapter to the eye (vision) and the ear (audition) with a wee bit about smell (olfaction). Taste (gustation) is mentioned in the chapter on the digestive system, and touch (tactioception) is associated with the integumentary system.

### The Eye

*"So through the eyes love attains the heart:*
*For the eyes are the scouts of the heart..."*
—Guiraut de Bornelh, troubadour (1138-1215)

## Function

After the brain, the eye is the most complex organ in the human body. It is useful in nonverbal communication and to convey understanding as in, "I see what you are saying," or "We see eye to eye" (which indicates we are in complete agreement).

# Key Vocabulary
## Eye

There are two combining forms referring to the eye.

1. **Ophthalm/o** is the Greek-sourced combining form for the eye. (Warning: Pet peeve approaching! Please note that this word has two consonant digraphs: *ph* and *th*. It is correctly pronounced, "off-thal-mo.") Examples:

**ophthalm/o/logy**   The study of disorders and treatments of the eye.

**ophthalm/o/scope**   The suffix **-scope** tells us that this is the instrument used in examining the interior of the eye.

**xer/ophthalm/ia** Pertaining to the condition of dry eyes.

**ophthalm/o/pleg/ia** Pertaining to paralysis of an eye.

2. **Ocul/o** is from the Latin meaning eye. Examples:

**ocul/ar/ist**   Specialist in the making and fitting of artificial eyes.

**intra/ocul/ar** Pertaining to within the eye.

**bin/ocul/ar**   Having to do with both eyes as in a binocular microscope, or opera glasses, or binoculars.

## Sight/Vision

The combining forms meaning sight or vision are **opt/o** and **vis/o**.

1. **Opt/o** is from the Greek. Examples:
   **optic/ian**   A person who makes and supplies eyeglasses and contact lenses as well as other optical instruments perhaps.
   **optic/o/kinet/ic**   Having to do with the movement of the eye.
   **opt/o/metr/ist**   A specialist, literally, in the measurement (**metr**) of the eye. The optometrist provides primary vision care, has a doctor of optometry degree, and is not a medical doctor (unlike an ophthalmologist).

2. **Vis/o** is from the Latin.

In the USA, students speak of studying or reviewing for an exam. In England, a student revises. Americans usually use "revise" to mean reconsider, alter, update, or improve. Now, both are correct; the words are synonyms. They both descend from the Latin verb *videre,* meaning to see. The prefix **re-** makes it "to see again." Other related descendants are visor, **vision**, television, visual.

The suffix **-opia** or **-opsia** means vision and is found in words like:
   **asthen/opia**   The word root here means lacking in strength or weak. The word means eyestrain.
   **dipl/opia**   Double vision.

**hyper/opia**   The condition of farsightedness.

**nyctal/opia**   The inability to see in dim light or night blindness.

**my/opia**   Commonly called nearsightedness.

**emmetr/opia**   Normal eyesight; the combining form **emmetr/o** means in correct measure.

## Iris

**Iris** is the name of the rainbow-hued goddess who was the messenger of the gods and whose name has been given to the colored part of the eye.

## Lens

There are two combining forms referring to the lens in the eye: **phac/o** or **phak/o**, and **lenticu/o** or **lent/o.**

1. **Phac/o** or **phak/o** come from the Greek. Examples:
   **phak/oma**   A very small (in fact, microscopic) tumor in the retina; the suffix **-oma** means tumor or mass.
   **a/phak/ia**   The condition of being without a lens.
   **phac/o/pathy**   An inclusive term for diseases of the lens.

2. **Lenticul/o** or **lent/o** come from the Latin. Examples:
   **lenticul/ar**   Shaped like a lens, or pertaining to a lens.
   **lent/o/pathy**   An inclusive term for disease conditions of the eye.

## Pupil

There are two combining forms referring to the pupil of the eye: **cor/o** and **pupill/o.**

1. **Cor/o** is from the Greek. Example:

**an/iso/cor/ia**   Do you remember isoceles triangles from math classes?   Recall their chief characteristic, and you will have the meaning of **is/o.** Is/o means equal. And the **iso**sceles triangle has equal sides. They are **iso**metric. A few years ago, I had a routine dilated eye exam. The next  morning, I awoke to a sense that my vision was not quite normal. A look in the bathroom mirror, and I got quite a fright: one **pupil** was of normal size, the other significantly larger. It was anisocordia, a condition of unequal pupils. A temporary condition, fortunately for me, just long enough for the dilating substance to completely drain from the eye.

2. **Pupill/o** is from the Latin and refers to the pupil of the eye.

### Eyelash

**Cili/um** refers to the eyelash. Just one. The plural is **cilia**. A person with a supercilious attitude is haughty, arrogant. It seems their eyebrow (or brows, **cili**) are raised (**super**) almost to their hairline.

### Eyelid

There are two combining forms that refer to the eyelid: **palpebr/o** and **blephar/o**.

1. **Palpebr/o** comes to us from the Latin. Example:
**palpebrate**  To blink or wink; not to be confused with **palpate** (to examine by touch) or **palpitate** (a rapid, pounding heartbeat).

2. **Blephar/o** comes to us from the Greek. Examples:

**blephar/o/spasm**     A twitching or involuntary contraction of the eyelid.

**blephar/o/ptosis** A condition of a drooping eyelid; the suffix, -**ptosis,** means drooping, sagging, prolapse.

### Tears

There are two combining forms referring to the tears we shed: **dacry/o** and **lacrim/o**.

1. The Greek *dakryon,* meaning tear, is the source for **dacry/o.** Examples:

**dacry/o/hem/o/rrhea**     Tears containing blood; the suffix -**rrhea** means flow or discharge.

**dacry/o/aden/algia**   Pain in a lacrimal gland.

**dacry/o/stenosis**   The condition of a narrowing of a tear duct.

2. The Latin *lacrima* also translates as tear and is the source of the combining form **lacrim/o**.  Examples:

**lachry/phag/y**   Literally, the eating of tears, but here it refers to drinking. Both the butterfly and the bee drink the tears of the crocodile (yes, crocodile tears) and are among other insects who feed on tears. The suffix -**y** means condition. (Notice the variation in the spelling of this word and the one below.)

**lachrym/ose**     One who is tearful; the suffix -**ose** means to be full of.

**lacrim/ation**   The secretion and discharge of tears.

## Cornea

There are two combining forms referring to the cornea in the eye.

1. **Kerat/o** is from the Greek. Examples:
    **kerat/o/plasty**   The suffix **-plasty** means a surgical repair, and in this case usually refers to a **corneal transplant.**
    **kerat/o/tomy**   The making of an incision (**-tomy**) into the cornea.

2. **Corne/o** is from the Latin. Examples:
    **corne/al**   Pertaining to the cornea
    **corne/o/blepharon**   Adhesion of the eyelid to the cornea.

## Additional Vocabulary

**Aqueous humor** is a watery fluid (**humor**) found in the anterior chamber of the eye. *Aqua* is the Latin word for water.

**OD** is the abbreviation for **oculus dexter,** meaning right eye. (It also is the abbreviation for overdose. which brings up an issue about abbreviations: they can be very confusing, and even dangerous, in medical situations. The context is a clue to the meaning, but if there is a possibility of misunderstanding, write out the whole word or phrase.)

**OS** stands for **oculus sinister** or left eye. The words **dexter** and **sinister** are an example of how prejudice gets encoded in words and carried down through time. **Dexter** means right. Look up the word "dexterous" in a dictionary and you will find adjectives like adroit, skillful, clever, artful, deft, and expert. **Sinister** (left) comes down to us directly in our word "sinister." Look that word up and you find adjectives like unlucky, unfavorable, evil, ill omen, trouble, and disaster. My mother went to school at a time when it was still not permitted for students to write with the left hand. She was a "southpaw" (south and left are sometimes connected as are right and north) and had to learn to write with her right hand. Between school and a right-handed mother teaching her to quilt, my mother was quite **ambi/dextr/ous**, the prefix **ambi-** meaning on both sides.

**OU** is the abbreviation for **oculus uterque,** referring to each eye or both eyes.

**Rods** and **cones** are the two types of photoreceptor (sensitive to, receptive to light) cells found in the eye. The rods are limited to perceiving only black and white shades while the cones perceive color. (My students found it helpful to remember this difference by thinking of the two which start with the same letter: cones and color.)

**Vitr/o** means glass as in **in vitro fertilization (IVF)**, the fertilization of an egg by a sperm in a glass petri dish, test tube, or some such laboratory container. Because our focus here is the eye, we can turn our attention to the **vitreous humor**, which is found in the posterior chamber of the eye. The adjective "vitreous" tells us that it is clear, transparent, like glass, and the word "humor" harkens back to the early Greek theory of humors or humours. An ophthalmologist once told me that, while the vitreous humor is gelatinous when we are young, as we age it becomes more like runny egg whites. Everything starts to sag, even the vitreous humor inside our eyes... Sigh.

## Maladies and Unwellnesses

The **Snellen eye chart** was named for Hermann Snellen, a Dutch ophthalmologist (1834-1908). It measures visual acuity and, with that big E at the top, is a familiar sight to many.

**A/stigmat/ism** is an imperfection in the curvature of the eye that results in blurred vision.

**Chalazion** is Greek for lump and refers to the localized swelling found at the edge of an eyelid and caused by obstruction of a **meibomian gland**. Not to be confused with a **hordeolum** (so much fun to say), which is caused by an infection of a **meibomian gland** and is commonly called a **sty.**

**Cataract** comes from the Greek *kato,* meaning down, and *raktos,* meaning precipice. A cataract is a synonym for a waterfall or a steep rapids. Looking at life through a cataract-clouded lens in the eye has been compared to looking through a rain-drenched window pane.

**Con/junctiv/itis** is an inflammation of the **conjunctiva**. The **conjunctiva** is the mucus membrane that lines the inside of the eyelid and covers the front of the eye. You may recognize this condition by its more common name, pinkeye.

**Ec/trop/ion** and **en/trop/ion** are two opposite conditions: in **ec/trop/ion** the eyelid —usually the lower lid—turns (**trop**) outward (**ec-**) and sags away from the eye. In **en/trop/ion,** the eyelid turns inward (**en-**), so that the eyelashes rub against the eye. The suffix **-ion** means process: the process of turning inward or outward.

**Glaucoma** is a condition of increased **intra/ocul/ar** pressure which can cause damage to the optic nerve. **Intra/ocul/ar** pertains to within the eye.

**Mio/sis** is an abnormal contraction of the pupils. (This term is a perfect homophone for—it sounds exactly the same as—**meio/sis**, the term for the cell division that forms the **gametes**. We'll meet up with the **gametes** when we talk about human reproduction.)

**Mydria/sis** is a condition (**-sis**) of a dilated pupil; it might be unilateral (pertaining to being one-sided) or non-isometric (pertaining to not equal in measurement).

**Macular degeneration** is a **chronic** (long-lasting) condition marked by the degeneration of the **macula**. The macula is found in the center of the retina.

**Nyct/al/opia** is the inability to see in dim light, also known as night blindness. **Nyct** has to do with night, **al** with blindness, and **-opia** with vision. Writing around 30 CE, Celsus, a Roman encyclopedist, had this to say about the condition: "There is a certain weakness of the eyes in which people see well in the daytime but not at all at night. This condition does not exist in women whose menstruation is regular. Those who suffer with this disability should anoint their eyeballs with the drippings from a liver while it is roasting—preferably that of a he-goat; if that is not possible, one from a she-goat; and the liver itself should be eaten." Interestingly, one of the causes of nyctalopia is a deficiency of vitamin A, found in the liver among other sources.

In the chapter on the nervous system, the term **photo/ phobia** is listed with the phobias, but it can also refer to having a sensitivity to light. This sensitivity is associated with such conditions as migraine, measles, rubella, meningitis, and inflammations of the eye.

**Presby/o** is a combining form with which I am increasingly familiar. It means old or elder. One may wonder, as I did on first contact, what old age has to do with the Protestant denomination called the Presbyterians. Then the enlightening struck. I remembered that Presbyterians are governed by a Presbytery, a council of elders. A presbyter is an elder in the church. Elders are the equivalent of bishops in some other Christian groups. And so, we have **presby/opia**, pertaining to old eyes or vision.

Besides being a spelling challenge, **pterygium** indicates the presence of a **benign** (non-cancerous) growth of excess tissue over the **sclera** (the white of the eye).

**Strabismus** is an abnormal alignment of the eyes, commonly called crossed eyes.

### The Ear

*"The most important thing in communication is hearing what isn't said."*
—Peter Drucker (1909–2005)

### Function

The term for the sense of hearing is **audition**. That's the same word that is used when one tries out for a part in a play. Does one go to get a hearing?

In addition to the sense of hearing, the ear also is involved in reporting to the brain on body movement and positioning or equilibrium.

## Key Vocabulary
### Ear

There are two combining forms referring to the ear: **ot/o** and **aur/o**.

1. The combining form **ot/o** comes from the Greek. Examples:

**ot/algia**   Pain in the ear, an earache.

**ot/itis media**   An inflammation in the ear; **media** indicates that the inflammation is in the middle ear.

**ot/o/myc/osis**  A condition of fungus in the ear, a fungal ear infection; sometimes known as swimmer's ear.

**ot/o/py/o/rrhea**   A discharge from the ear that contains pus.

**ot/o/rrhea**  Any discharge from the ear.

2. **Aur/o** comes from the Latin and means ear. Examples:

**aur/icle**   The outer ear, handy for piercing and sometimes the subject of teasing. Another name for this appendage is the **pinna** or **pinnae** if referring to more than one. The combining form is **pinn/i**, and it comes from the Latin meaning wing. This term is also found in zoology where it refers to a feather, wing, fin, or other similarly shaped body part or appendage. As a small child, I remember how much I hated helping my grandmother pluck a chicken, and especially the pin feathers! Now, watching her catch the chicken (after dark when the chickens were asleep in their coop), and twist its neck or behead it, that was more fascinating. Once, when one got away, I learned first-hand what the saying "running around like a chicken with its head cut off" really looked like.

**auri/form**   In the shape of an ear.

**auris dextra**   The right ear.

**auris sinistra**   The left ear.

## Hearing

There are two combining forms which refer to hear or hearing.

1. **Acous/o** or **acoust/o** is from the Greek. Examples:
   **acoust/ic**   Pertaining to the sense of hearing; in contemporary music, it refers to not having electrical amplification. Acoustics, as a noun, refers to the properties or qualities of a room that make hearing sounds easy or difficult.
   **acoust/ic/o/phobia**   An abnormal fear of loud noises.

2. **aud/i, aud/o** or **audit/o** are from the Latin. Examples:
   **Audi**   the name of an automobile.
   **audible**   Able to be heard in an auditorium, a large building or hall where concerts or speeches are heard; to audit a class is to attend (hear) the class but not receive academic credit.
   **aud/o/meter**   An instrument used to test hearing.
   **audi/o/gen/ic**   Pertaining to originating in sound.

## Cochlea

**Cochlea** is a spiral cavity in the inner ear. The spiral is a common pattern in nature, seen in galaxies and snail shells: *cochlea* is the Latin word for snail shell. The Greek word is similar: *kokhlos.*

## Eustachian Tube

The **eustachian tube** extends from the throat to the middle ear. The combining form **salping/o** refers both to the **eustachian tube** and the **fallopian tube** (which we will discuss in the chapter on the reproductive system).

## Labyrinth

**Labyrinth/o:** A labyrinth is a recognizable pattern that has been around since ancient times, at least back to the Minoan civilization on Crete, and today we still have mazes or labyrinths used for walking meditation. The labrys or double ax is a common Minoan symbol for a goddess. In the ear, it gives its name to a complex structure in the inner ear.

## Auditory Ossicles

**Malleus, incus, stapes:** These are the **auditory ossicles** or little bones. The word **malleus** means hammer. In 1486, a book was written titled *Malleus Maleficarum* (*The Hammer of Witches*). Its authors, Heinrich Kramer and Jacob Sprenger, promoted the persecution of witches and the eradication of witchcraft. They died; Wicca lives. Just saying... **Incus** is Latin for anvil and **stapes** for stirrup. The stapes is the smallest bone in the body and is about the size of a grain of rice.

## Mastoid Process

**Mastoid process** (**mast/oid** means resembling a female breast) is a rounded, downward pointing, bony projection of the skull near the ears.

## Eardrum

There are two combining forms for the eardrum.

1. **Tympan/o** comes from the Greek. Examples:
   **tympani**   In drums and eardrums.
   **tympan/o/centesis**   The suffix **-centesis** refers to a surgical puncture—to remove fluid, in this case from the middle ear, behind the eardrum.
   **tympan/o/scler/osis**   A condition in which hard fibrous tissue grows around the ossicles of the middle ear.

2. **Myring/o** comes to us from the Latin. Examples:
   **myring/o/tomy**   A cut or incision is made into the eardrum.
   **myring/ectomy**      The excision or removal of the tympanic membrane.

## Sound

**Phon/o** is the combining form for sound. There are lots of examples in words which are in everyday usage:
   **symphony**      Literally, the process of sounding together.
   **polyphony**   Many or a variety of sounds.
   **cacophony**   *Kakos* in Greek means bad; cacophony is a harsh, clamorous mixture of sounds.
   **telephone**   Tele- means far.

**phonograph** Literally, writer of sounds.

**euphony** or **euphonious** The opposite of cacophony, it means sounding good, agreeable. What is the most euphonious sound in your life?

**phonetics** Pertaining to sound; it is the scientific study of speech.

I'll offer one medical example:

**dysphonia** Hoarseness of voice or difficulty in speaking.

### Additional Vocabulary

**Auscultation** literally means the act of listening; in medicine, it is the use of a **stethoscope** to listen for sounds within the body, for example, in the abdomen or the lungs.

**Cerumen** is the medical term for earwax (the Latin *cera* means wax).

### Maladies and Unwellnesses

**An/acu/sis** is a condition of no hearing; a loss of hearing.

**Hyper/acu/sis** is abnormally acute hearing.

**Meniere's disease** is a disorder of the inner ear that causes spontaneous episodes of **vertigo**, fluctuating **anacusis**, **tinnitus,** and sometimes feelings of pressure in the ear.

**Ot/o/rhin/o/laryng/o/logy** is the study of the ear, the nose, and the throat—although the **larynx** is the voice box, and the **pharynx** is the throat. Hmmm.

**Par/ot/itis** is an inflammation of the **parotid gland**; **par-** means near or alongside, and **ot** means ear.

**Presby/cu/sis** refers to the hearing of the elderly (**presby**); a gradual hearing loss as people age.

**Tinnitus** is a ringing in the ears and comes from one of my favorite words to say: *tintinnabulum*. It just rolls off the tongue. It is the Latin word for tinkling bell. The play and movie, *A Funny Thing Happened on the Way to the Forum*, has a character named Tintinnabula. It was fun to hear from a former student that she had played this role in her high school production. Needless to say, she had no trouble with this vocabulary word. The Latin infinitive *tinnire* means to ring or tinkle.

**Vertigo** means dizziness. *Vertigo* is a Latin word that originally meant a whirling or spinning movement.

### And Finally...
### Smell

*"The first condition of understanding a foreign country is to smell it."*
—Rudyard Kipling (1865–1936)

**Olfaction** is the sense of smell. Some relevant terms are listed below:

**Rhin/o** is the combining form for the nose. Think rhinoceros. A **rhin/o/plasty** is a nose job; the surgical repair of the nose.

**Mal/odor/ous** pertains to a bad smell.

**An/osm/ia** pertains to having no smell, a loss of the sense of smell. The root **osme** means smell or odor.

I sense another chapter approaching...

# Chapter Eight
## The Respiratory System

*"It was the fashion to suffer from the lungs; everybody was consumptive, poets especially; it was good form to spit blood after any emotion that was at all sensational, and to die before reaching the age of thirty."*
—Alexandre Dumas, fils (1824-95)

## Introduction

The respiratory system is comprised of the nose, where the action starts with air entering the body from our external environment; then come the nasal sinuses, pharynx, larynx, trachea, bronchi, bronchioles, and the alveoli, where gas exchange occurs with the capillaries of the bloodstream. This system first functions at birth with that first intake of air, allowing the newborn to cry and the parent(s) to breathe a sigh of relief.

## Function

The goal of the respiratory system is to bring oxygen from that air we just inhaled and get it to the bloodstream, which will pick up the job of supplying the body's cells with this essential component. And then, in a most efficient manner, the waste product, carbon dioxide, is removed from the body when we breathe out. In another display of efficiency, this process produces the airflow that moves over the larynx and makes speech possible.

## Key Vocabulary
### Oxygen

**Ox/o** is the combining form for oxygen. The suffix **-oxia** and the prefix **oxy-** also refer to this important element. *Oxys* in the Greek means sharp, acid.

When Joseph Priestley identified this element in England in 1774, he called it "dephlogisticated air" (it's a long story involving phlogiston theory). It was Antoine-Laurent Lavoisier, a French chemist, who noted in 1775 that all the acids he worked with contained this same element. Because he thought it was an acid producer, he named it **oxy/gen,** meaning to produce or form acid. Oxydol and Oxiclean are examples of the use of this word part. Medspeak gives us these examples:

**an/ox/ic** Pertaining to being without, lacking oxygen.
**hyp/ox/ic** Pertaining to being deficient in oxygen.

### Breath and Breathing

There are two combining forms meaning breath: **pne/o** and **hal/o**.

1. *Pneuma* is Greek for breath. In philosophy, it refers to the soul, the vital spirit, one's creative force. The combining

form for use in medical terms is **pne/o,** and the suffix is **-pnea**. You will find a variety of words using this suffix later on in this chapter. You will also note, when we come to the words meaning lung, that a closely related combining form, **pneum/o,** can mean air or lung.

2. From the Latin, we get **hal/o** for breath. Perhaps you have heard of or experienced **halit/osis**, literally, a condition of the breath and in common usage bad breath. **In/hale, ex/hale, in/hal/ation,** and **ex/hal/ation** are examples using this word root.

The combining form **spir/o,** from the Greek, perhaps comes the closest to merging the mechanics of breathing with the mystery of the spirit of life. **In/spir/ation** is a synonym for **in/hal/ation**: to draw breath in. We also use it when talking about creativity and motivation. To **ex/pire** is to **ex/hale**, to breathe out, and also to die, the departing of spirit from the body.

To **a/spir/ate** is to draw in or out by suction, as in a parent **a/spir/ating** mucus from an infant's airway or someone aspirating foreign objects into their lungs. While one's **aspiration** is one's goal, dream or yearning hope, it is also a condition, as in **aspiration pneumonia**.

**Re/spir/ation** is to breathe again and again, repeated **inspirations** and **expirations**, the prefix **re-** meaning again as in to repeat.

There are actually **two respiratory processes** occurring within our bodies. The one we are conscious of is **external respiration** or **ventilation** (as in when one **hyper/ventilates**) and involves **inspiration** and **expiration**. The other process, **internal respiration**, involves the exchange of gases (oxygen and carbon dioxide) at a cellular level.

The next grouping of key words relates to the anatomy of the respiratory system.

### Nose

Both **nas/o** and **rhin/o** are combining forms that refer to the nose.

1. The combining form **nas/o** comes to us from the Latin. Examples:
    **nas/al**  Pertaining to the nose.
    **nas/o/gastr/ic**  Pertaining to the nose and stomach; a **nas/o/gastr/ic** tube passes through the nose into the stomach.

2. **Rhin/o** is from the Greek. Examples:
    **rhino/tillexis**  A compulsive picking of the nose.
    **rhin/itis**  Inflammation of the nose, perhaps due to the common cold or an allergic reaction.
    **rhin/o/rrhea**  Nasal discharge, a runny nose accompanying a **rhin/itis**.

### Nasal Sinuses

**Sinus/o**  A **sinus** is a cavity.

### Pharynx

**Pharyng/o** is the combining form for the, **pharynx** which is commonly called the throat. Examples:

**pharyng/itis** A sore throat; an inflammation of the throat.
**pharyng/o/tomy** An incision into the pharynx; the suffix **-tomy** means to cut into, incise.

## Larynx

The **larynx** (combining form **laryng/o**) is commonly known as the voice box. It is part of the air passage to the lungs. The flow of air over the vocal cords produces sound.

## Trachea

Trachea (**trache/o**) is commonly referred to as the windpipe. Examples:
**trache/o/tomy** An incision or cut made to relieve an obstruction to breathing.
**trache/o/stomy** The surgical creation of a new opening. **Stoma** in medspeak refers to a mouth or opening. The **trache/o/stomy** is meant to be more permanent than the **trache/o/tomy**.

## Bronchi

**Bronchus** and the plural **bronchi** come from the Greek *bronkhos,* meaning windpipe. The **bronchi** are found in the lungs and are airways that resemble a tree. The twigs are called **bronchioles**.

## Alveoli

**Alveol/o** is the combining form for the **alveolus** (plural **alveoli**), which is a tiny air sac found in the lung—multiplied by 300 million, give or take a few.

# Additional Vocabulary
## Lungs

There are two combining forms for the lungs: **pneum/o** or **pneumon/o** and **pulmon/o**.

1. From the Greek, we get **pneum/o** or **pneumon/o**. Examples:

**pneum/o/gastr/ic**    Pertaining to the lungs and the stomach.

**pneumon/ia**    Literally, a condition of the lungs. It is one of a very few medical inflammatory conditions that do not use the suffix **-itis**. Another is **pleurisy,** which refers to an inflammation of the **pleura,** one of two membranes encasing the lungs.

**pneum/o/cele**    A hernia of the lung; the suffix **-cele** means hernia.

2. The combining form from the Latin is **pulmon/o**. Perhaps you have anticipated this example:

**pulmon/ary**    Pertaining to the lungs.

## Chest

There are three combining forms referring to the chest: **thorac/o**, **pector/o,** and **steth/o**.

1. The Greeks have given us the first two of the three: **thorac/o.** Examples:

**thorax**    The chest, the part of our body between the neck and the diaphragm.

**thorac/o/tomy**    A cut or incision in the chest.

2. The second, also from the Greek, is **pector/o.** Example:
**pector/al**   Pertaining to the chest.

3. The Latin contribution is **steth/o**. Example:
**steth/o/scope**      Literally, an instrument used to examine the chest.

## Diaphragm

**Phren/o** is the combining form for the diaphragm in this chapter. (In the chapter on the nervous system, you will find another definition for this combining form.) Examples:
**phren/algia** or **phren/o/dynia**   Pain in the diaphragm.
**phren/ic** Pertaining to the **diaphragm** or the **phrenic nerve**.

**Septum**, **parietal**, and the suffix **-phragm** all refer to a wall or partition.

## Pulse

*Sphygmos* is Greek for pulse, as we discovered in the chapter about the circulatory system. The combining form is **sphygm/o**. Another form of the word is *sphyxis,* as in the suffix **-sphyxia**. Examples:
**a/sphyx/ia**  Lack of a pulse. It has now come to mean a condition caused by insufficient intake of oxygen.
**a/sphyx/iate**  To suffocate, die due to lack of oxygen.

## Sputum

The word **sputum** comes from the Latin *spuere,* meaning to spit. Sputum is defined as a secretion thicker than ordinary spittle or saliva.

## Glottis and Epiglottis

**Epiglott/o** is the combining form for the **epi/glottis**. The **glottis** consists of the vocal cords and the opening between them. The **epiglottis** is a flap of cartilage that folds over and protects the entrance to the **larynx** during swallowing—it keeps food from "going down the wrong way." Note the prefix **epi-** in **epiglottis,** which means above or upon.

## Bonus Word

**Oscitation** is the act of yawning.

## Maladies and Unwellnesses

**Agon/al** breathing is related to death or dying. The Greek *agon* means contest. Originally referring to a struggle for victory in an athletic contest, it was only later that it became associated with extreme bodily suffering preceding death.

**Asthma** comes directly from the Greek *asthma,* meaning to pant.

**Atel/ectasis:** The word root **atel** comes from the Greek *ateles*, meaning not perfect. The suffix **-ectasis** refers to expansion. This word describes a lung that has collapsed and is airless, or a lung that at birth either does not expand or only partially expands.

**Coryza** comes from the Greek meaning catarrh. Commonly referred to as the common cold. **Catarrh** is the inflammation of the mucus membranes, characterized by excessive secretions.

**Croup** is an acute viral disease usually found in the pediatric crowd. Its chief characteristic is a cough that has been described as sounding like a barking seal; it is worse when one is lying down.

**Emphysema** is a chronic, progressive lung disease and part of the group of conditions referred to as **COPD**, **chronic obstructive pulmonary disease**.

**Epi/staxis** comes from the Greek meaning to drop or drip upon and, appropriately, is the term for nosebleed.

**Expectorant** is an agent (**-ant**), a medicine in this case, that helps get rid of (**ex-**) sputum from the chest (**pector**).

**Hemo/ptysis** is bloody sputum. **Ptysis** means spit—and when saying this word one has to be very careful not to spray spit on those in the immediate area.

**Hyper/capnia** describes an abnormal increase of carbon dioxide in the body. **Capn/o** is the combining form for carbon dioxide.

---

**Influenza** is usually shortened to the flu and is a respiratory infection.

As a child, and into my adult years, I loved to jump rope. For your diversion, I offer a poem that my father taught me and is sometimes used as an accompaniment for jumping rope:

> I had a little bird
> Its name was Enza
> I opened the window
> And in-flu-enza.

This little verse dates from the 1918 Spanish influenza pandemic through which my dad lived; perhaps that is when he learned it.

You may also hear among older folk the word **grippe** used as a synonym for the flu. **Grippe** is the French word for seizure.

---

**Nas/o/pharyng/itis** is an inflammation in the nose and the throat.

**Pertussis** is commonly known as whooping cough.

---

**Pneum/o/thorax:** These two word roots (**pneum/o** meaning air or lung and **thorac/o** meaning chest) tell us that there is air or gas in the chest, specifically the pleural cavity, where it should not be. There is a leak. There are two types of **pneumothoraces: spontaneous** and **traumatic.**

Here is a story to **illustrate the traumatic**: The all-female nursing school that I attended attracted students from around the USA and from different countries. It was common for us to go home with other students or invite others to our homes during any break time. And there was a lot of knitting going on at this school—mostly scarves or sweaters for boyfriends. So, in response to an assignment, several of my classmates and I came up with a skit in which we were traveling to someone's home, all knitting to pass the time. Except for the driver, of course. When we were involved in an accident, you guessed it, someone was stabbed in the chest with a knitting needle: a **traumatic pneumothorax**.

I have a more personal experience with a **spontaneous pneumothorax.** A few years after the anecdote recounted above, I was working at the University of Illinois Hospital in Chicago, and my husband of less than a year was a student at Northwestern University. One day, while taking an exam, he suddenly began to feel ill. This was not just nerves associated with the exam. He had a deep knowing that something was seriously not right. He left his class and drove his little red MGB convertible across campus to the student health center. As soon as the nurse saw him, she grabbed a wheelchair... or a gurney—I can't remember which. He was quickly transported to a hospital. I received a phone call in my office telling me that my husband was in the emergency room at Evanston Hospital and to get myself to the hospital ASAP. He was diagnosed with a **spontaneous pneumothorax**. There was no evident etiology—no cause, origin, or reason for this occurrence. Perhaps there had been a blister on the pleura that had burst. (And who knows how long he had already lived with that blister?) He might never have another occurrence, or he might, is what he was told. His lung collapsed again while he was recovering in the hospital. It was a rather harrowing time. I can report that thus far there has been no repeat performance. Thankfully!

## Pus

There are two combining forms for pus, **py/o** and **purul/o**.

1. **Py/o** comes from the Greek. Example:
   **py/o/thorax**   Tells us there is pus in the chest.

2. From the Latin, we have **purul/o**. Example:
   **purulent**   Tells us pus is present.

---

## Pnea

The word root **pnea** refers to the breath. There are a variety of descriptive words formed by adding the appropriate prefix.

**ana/pnea**   To regain one's breath.

**a/pnea**   Literally, to be without breath (the prefix **a-** or **an-** meaning no, not, without). It means a temporary cessation of breathing, as in **sleep apnea.**

**brady/pnea**   Slow breathing.

**dys/pnea**   Painful or difficult breathing.

**hyper/pnea**   Increased breath rate such as after exercise—or there may be a more serious cause.

**orth/o/pnea**   Literally, straight breathing. This person has difficulty breathing when lying down and needs to be sitting up.

**poly/pnea**   Many breaths, or panting.

**tachy/pnea**   Rapid breathing.

And saved for last:

**eu/pnea**   Normal breathing.

---

## All Is Well

The prefix **eu-** means well, good, normal, and can be found in such words as "eulogy," which literally means good words or to speak well of. A euphemism is auspicious, sounding good. Euphoria, the Eurythmics, the Eucharist (the root *kharis* in Greek means favor or grace). A euonym is a good or appropriate name, for example, a realtor might be named Betty House. To have eunomia is to have order; to have disnomia, disorder. Medical examples:

> **eucrasia**  Normal health; all activities (**-crasia** means mixture) are in balance.
> **eu/thyr/oid**  A normally functioning thyroid.
> **eu/thanas/ia**  Literally, pertaining to a good death. The Greek *thanatos* means death.

Eureka!

In **re/sus/cit/ate**, the word root **cit** comes from the Latin verb *citare,* meaning to put in motion, to rouse; **sus** means up from and **re-** means again.

*Stertere* is the Latin meaning to snore; **stertorous** refers to noisy, labored breathing.

**Thora/centesis:** The suffix **-centesis** indicates a surgical puncture, in this case, into the chest. This is usually for the purpose of withdrawing fluid for diagnostic purposes.

A **tonsill/ectomy** and an **adenoid/ectomy,** a **T&A** for short, was once a common childhood surgical procedure. The suffix **–ectomy** is defined as a surgical removal, excision, or resection. It was thought that removal would result in fewer throat and ear infections. I remember hearing people talk about children "getting to that age" when they would need to have their tonsils removed—it was something of a rite of passage. I also heard that some doctors would offer group or family rates when several children were close to the same age. "He/she is going to need them out anyway. Might as well do it now." I was six years old when my T&A was performed in our family doctor's office with his wife/ nurse administering the ether.

**Tubercul/osis** is an infectious disease commonly affecting the respiratory tract. An earlier name for tuberculosis was **consumption**, and earlier than that, **phthisis**. In the 1800s, when tuberculosis occurrences were near **epidemic** proportions in industrialized countries, treatment might include fresh air and jolting, as in a carriage ride on a country road. Or, a patient might stay in an airtight room wrapped in a blanket by a hot stove. When sanatoria, places designed for the care of patients with **TB**, came into being in the latter part of the nineteenth century, they were generally located in rural areas where fresh air and sunshine—and good food—were part of the prescriptive therapy. As student nurses, my classmates and I spent six weeks caring for patients at a TB sanatorium, where we lived in a dormitory. We were actually a bit sad to leave as the setting was so lovely and the food was better than at our home hospital!

### Bonus Section

Some people are fascinated with words and word trivia. I am. When I was about eleven years old, I discovered what I understood to be the longest word in the English language, "antidisestablishmentarianism." Ah, now there's a word you can get your tongue around!

But then I discovered a longer word! I immediately had to learn it. And it has medical connections! It is: **pneumonoultramicroscopicsilicovolcanokoniosis.**

Now, more recently, in a marketing piece for educational materials, I have seen an even longer version of this term, which has been elongated by adding a prefix: **intrapneumonoultramicroscopicsilicovolcanokoniosis.**

Here is a breakdown: **intra** (within), **pneumono** (lung), **ultra** (beyond), **micro** (small), **scopic** (pertaining to viewing), **silico** (silicon carbon), **volcano** (vent), **koni** (dust), and **osis** (condition). Taken all together, we have a lung disease caused by inhaling very fine dust particles, a condition found commonly in miners. Such excessively long words—sometimes artificially constructed—are not practical and are not usually found in everyday usage. It is enough to call the above simply **pneumonoconiosis**, which is long enough.

# Chapter Nine
## The Digestive System

*"Why should we not meet, not always as dyspeptics, to tell our bad dreams, but sometimes as eupeptics, to congratulate each other on the ever glorious morning? I do not make an exorbitant demand, surely."*
—Henry David Thoreau (1817–1862)

### Introduction

The digestive system is also known as the gastrointestinal (GI) tract and the alimentary canal. The word "alimentary" comes from the Latin *alimentum*, meaning nourishment. Food enters at the mouth, it is processed along the way, and the waste products leave the canal through the anus. Other words coming from the same ancient roots as alimentary are: "alimony" (a provision for sustenance or nourishment) and "alumnus/alumna" (nourished one, a pupil).

## Function

Ingestion, mastication, deglutition, absorption, and defecation. That sums it up! The purpose of the digestive system is to **ingest** (take food into the mouth) and **masticate** (chew); then follows **deglutition** (the act of swallowing), **absorption** (the various processes by which the body makes use of the nourishment provided), and finally **defecation** (discharge from the body). This conveyor belt for food, from mouth to anus, converts the food into a form that can be used by the body for energy, growth, and repair.

# Key Vocabulary
## Digestion

**Digest/ion** is the action, the process, by which foods are broken down into a form that can be used by the body. There are three combining forms here. The Latin combining form is the straightforward **digest/o**, while the Greek combining forms are the related **peps/o** and **pept/o.** These probably look familiar to you. Perhaps you have taken the pink Pepto Bismol for **dys/peps/ia**, the condition of a painful or difficult digestion. Or, perhaps you have taken a drink of Pepsi, a beverage originally created by a pharmacist and in early ads touted as a digestive aid. **Eu/peps/ia** tells us that all is well (**eu-**) in the digestion department.

## Metabolism

**Metabolism** is the collective name of the chemical processes that occur in the body to maintain life. **Metabolism** is made up of **anabolism**, the storing of energy (**ana-** has to do with building up) and **catabolism**, the releasing of energy (**cata-** has to do with breaking down). The origin of the word "catastrophe" is down (**cata**) turn (**trop**). Somewhat understated, considering its usage today, isn't it?

Following are the anatomical terms for this system beginning at the entry to the body.

## Lips

**Lip** has two combining forms: **cheil/o** and **labi/o**.

1. The Greek-based is **cheil/o**. Examples:
   **cheil/itis**   Inflammation of the lip.
   **cheil/o/rrhaphy**   Surgical repair (**-rrhaphy**) of the lip; used primarily to refer to repairing a cleft lip.

2. The Latin-based is **labi/o**. Examples:
   **labi/al/ism**   A type of stammering in which sounds made by the lips are prominent.
   **labi/o/dent/al**   Pertaining to the lips and the teeth.

## Mouth

The **mouth** has two combining forms: **stomat/o** and **or/o**.

1. The Greek combining form is **stomat/o**. (**Stoma** refers to the mouth; the plural of **stoma** is **stomata**.) Examples:
   **traumatic stomatitis**   Inflammation of the mouth brought about by something like ill-fitting dentures, a jagged-edged tooth, or biting the inside of the cheek.
   **stomat/o/gnath/ic**   Pertaining to both the mouth and the jaw (**gnath**).

**stomat/o/malacia**   The abnormal softening of any of the structures of the mouth.

2. The Latin gives us **or/o**. The Latin word **os** (plural **ora**) is used to mean mouth or opening. **Os** (plural **ossa**), also from the Latin, means bone. Use the context of the term to tell you whether it is bones or mouths under discussion. Examples:

**or/al**   Pertaining to the mouth, as in **oral hygiene**.
**or/o/lingu/al**   Pertaining to the mouth and the tongue.
**os uteri**   The mouth of the uterus.
**os/cul/ation**   The act of kissing.

### Dental Terms

Now that we are inside the mouth, terminologically speaking, let's learn some words relevant to the world of dentistry.

The **apex** of the tooth is the tip of the root.

**Bruxism** is the condition (**-ism**) of grinding, gnashing, or clenching of the teeth.

**Buccal** refers to the cheeks or mouth cavity as in the buccal side of the molars. *Bucca* is Latin for cheek.

**Gums:** One dental hygiene product in my medicine cabinet says that it helps fight gum disease, and another states that it is an **anti/gingiv/itis** product. They are saying the same thing, as **gingiv/o** is the combining form for the gum. With **-itis** meaning inflammation and **anti-** meaning against, we have two products declaring their fight against gum disease.

## Tooth/teeth

There are two combining forms for teeth: **dent/i** and **odont/o**.

1. From the Latin comes **dent/i**. Examples:
    **dent/i/frice**  A paste or powder for cleaning the teeth; **frice** comes from the Latin infinitive *fricare*, meaning to rub—think "friction."
    **dentin**  The hard substance in teeth under the enamel.
    **dent/ist**  One who specializes in teeth.
    **labi/o/dent/al**  Pertaining to the lips (**labi/o**) and teeth (**dent**).

2. From the Greek comes **odont/o**. Examples:
    **end/odont/ia**  A condition within (**endo**) the tooth. This is the term for anything having to do with the dental pulp found within the tooth. Commonly it is called a root canal.
    **orth/odont/ia**  The condition of straight teeth.
    **peri/odont/al**  Pertaining to around the tooth.

## Surfaces of the Tooth

The surface of a lower tooth, which faces inward towards the tongue, is called the **lingual** side. On the upper teeth, the inner aspect is called the **palatal.** That side facing outward—the side people see—is the **buccal**, as it is closer to the cheek. The side facing towards the front of the mouth is the **mesial** (**mes/o** means middle), and the surface facing towards the back is the **distal**. The **incisal** surface is the biting edge of the anterior teeth. The biting surface of the posterior teeth is the **occlusal**. The upper teeth are referred to as the **maxillary**, as in the **maxilla** or upper jaw. The bottom teeth are the **mandibular,** which refers to the **mandible**, the lower jawbone.

To have a dental **caries** is to have a cavity. *Caries* is the Latin for rottenness or decay.

To **articulate** in dentistry is to arrange teeth on a denture.

A **dental esthetician** is concerned with the appearance of a dental restoration.

### Elsewhere in the Mouth
### Tongue

There are two combining forms meaning **tongue: gloss/o** and **lingu/o**.

1. The Greek gives us **gloss/o.** Examples:
   **gloss/o/trich/ia**   Literally, the condition of a hairy (**trich**) tongue.
   **gloss/o/plegia**  Pertaining to a paralysis of the tongue.
   **gloss/o/lalia**  The ability to speak in another language without having learned it; "speaking in tongues," perhaps as part of a religious practice.

2. The Latin gifts us with **lingu/o.** Examples:
   **sub/lingu/al**  Pertaining to under the tongue. Certain pills or tablets are absorbed into the body by placing them under the tongue. **Sub/gloss/al** works as well.
   **ingu/o/gingiv/al**   Pertaining to the tongue and the gums (**gingiv/o**).

## Saliva

**Saliva** has its two ancient roots as well: **sial/o** and **saliv/o**.

1. **Sial/o** is from the Greek. Examples:
   **sial/o/lith**   A stone (**lith/o**) in a **salivary** gland.
   **sial/o/aden/o/tomy**   An incision has been made into a salivary gland.

2. **Saliv/o** comes from the Latin. Do you notice how frequently the Latin root has come down to us unchanged? Examples:
   **saliv/ary**   Pertaining to saliva.
   **saliv/ation**   The excess secretion of saliva. Just thinking about a lemon will activate the process.

## Let's Rejoin the GI Tract
## Esophagus

The **esophagus** has for its combining form **esophag/o**.

## Stomach

The combining form for the **stomach** is **gastr/o**. Gastronomy is the art of choosing, cooking, and eating food. Medical examples:
   **gastr/o/esophag/eal reflux disease**   Abbreviated **GERD**, this is a digestive disorder.
   **gastr/o/enter/o/col/itis**   An inflammation of the stomach, small intestine, and colon.
   **gastr/o/enter/o/logist**   A specialist in the study of the stomach and the small intestine.
   **gastr/o/scope**   An instrument used to visually examine the stomach.

## Abdomen

The **abdomen** has three combining forms.

1. The Greeks have given us two: **celi/o** and **lapar/o**. Examples:
    **celi/ac**   Pertaining to the abdomen.
    **celi/oma**   A tumor (**-oma**) of the abdomen.
    **lapar/o/tomy**   An incision into the abdomen; **celi/o/tomy** is a synonym. An **exploratory lapar/o/tomy** is a diagnostic operation done to examine the **abdomin/al** organs.
    **lapar/o/rrhaphy**   The suturing of the **abdomin/al** wall, perhaps to repair a wound.

2. The Latin root is the direct antecedent for **abdomin/o**. Example:
    **abdomin/al**   Pertaining to the abdomen; a synonym for **celi/ac**.

## Intestinal Terms

**Intestine** has two combining forms: **enter/o** and **intestin/o**.

1. The combining form from the Greek is **enter/o,** which, in common usage, is often used to specify the small intestine. In addition to the examples given above, I add:
    **enter/ic-coated**   The suffix (**-ic**) tells us that this term means pertaining to the intestine.

2. The Latin-based combining form is **intestin/o.**

A synonym for the intestine is **bowel**. Bowel comes from the Latin *bolulus*, meaning sausage.

The **duodenum** comes first. **Duodenum** is Latin for the number twelve, as in twelve finger breadths in length, which is what our ancients measured it to be. (The use of body parts as a unit of measure is illustrated by measuring the height of horses in hands.)

**Jejunum** means empty in Latin. This section of the intestine always seemed to be empty when the ancients examined it during a dissection.

**Ileum**—*ileos* in Latin—means severe colic; while *eileos* in the Greek means rolling or twisting. This is the third section of the small intestine. Don't confuse this word with the **ilium**, the pelvic bone!

**Cecum** comes from the Latin *caecum*, which means blind or hidden; the cecum is a blind pouch at the juncture of the small and large intestine.

**Colon** is the term for the large intestine, comprised of the **ascending**, **transverse** and **descending colon**. When the area of the body affected by a medical condition involves both the **colon** and the **rectum**, the term used is **colorectal**.

> **Q:** What is the term for half of the large intestine?
> **A:** A semi-colon!
> (Feel free to boo!)

**Sigmoid** comes from the Greek *sigma* and **-oid**, the suffix which means resembling. This section of the colon was so named for its resemblance to the Greek letter *s* (the *sigma*) and it leads into the rectum.

**Rectum** is from the Latin meaning straight as in erect. **Rectalgia**? A pain in the butt.

From the Greek we get the combining form **proct/o**, which refers to both the anus and the rectum, as in **proct/o/logist** (the specialist in all things **rectal** and **anal**) or **proct/itis**, an inflammation of the **rectal/anal** area.

The combining form for **anus** is **an/o** which comes to us from the Latin referring to a ring or sphincter of muscle.

### Additional Vocabulary

**Appendix** comes to us from the Latin verb *appendere* meaning "to cause to hang." In the human body the appendix hangs onto the intestine, while the appendix of a book hangs onto the main body of the work. **Vermiform appendix** is the full name of this dangling tissue found in humans. "Vermiform" means shaped like a worm. Vermicelli is a long slender pasta.

---

**Bile** is a bitter fluid secreted by the liver. It has two combining forms, **chol/e** and **bil/i**:

**chol/e** from the Greek. Examples:

**chol/e/stasis**   Tells us that the flow of bile from the liver has been arrested or is standing still (**stasis**).

**Chol/e/lith/iasis**   The condition of gallstones; **lith/o** means stone. **Gall** is another name for **bile.**

**chol/e/cyst/ectomy**   The surgical removal, excision, of the gall (**chole**) bladder (**cyst**).

**bil/i** from the Latin *bilis* means bile. Examples:
   **bili/ary**   The suffix **-ary** means pertaining to; thence, the term means pertaining to bile.
   **bili/genesis**   The formation of bile.

---

A **bolus** is a lump or ball of chewed food all ready to be swallowed.

**Catharsis** comes from the Greek word for a cleansing, and a **cathartic** is a type of medication that causes the bowel to empty, a purgative.

**Chyme,** from the Greek for juice, consists of gastric juices and partially digested food as it passes from the stomach into the small intestine. Chyme is related to a term found in the chapter on the integumentary system: **ecchymosis**, where the juice referred to is blood. **Chyle**, a word derived from the same Greek root, consists of a mixture of lymph and fats found in the intestinal tract during the digestion of fatty foods.

---

### Fats

There are two combining forms for fats: **steat/o** and **lip/o**.

1. The Greek-based combining form is: **steat/o**. Example:
   **steat/o/pygia**   An abnormal fatness of the buttocks.

2. The Latin is **lip/o**. Example:
   **lip/o/suction**   A procedure to remove fat tissue that is **sub/cutane/ous** or **sub/derm/al** (under the skin).

---

**Gustation** is the action of tasting and comes from the Latin *gustare,* meaning to taste. To feel "disgust" means to have a distaste for, to feel revulsion for, to be repelled by, sickened, "put off food." "Gusto" means an appetite for life.

**Hemorrhoids** are swollen veins in the area of the **anus**. Sometimes you will hear this condition called **piles**.

**Laxative,** which comes from the Latin *laxare,* meaning to loosen, is a substance which causes the bowel or stool to loosen and be passed from the body more readily. Have you heard it said that someone has lax work habits? They have loosened or slackened their standards.

**Pancreas** is a word derived from the Greek *pan,* meaning all or entire, and *kreas,* meaning flesh. The pancreas is entirely constituted of flesh without muscular tissues. Anatomists as early as Aristotle and Galen were using this term. This organ secretes digestive juices and the hormones insulin and glucagon.

**Peristalsis** comes from the Greek: **peri,** which means surrounding (as in perimeter) and **stalsis,** which means constriction. **Peristalsis** is the wavelike alternating contraction and relaxation of muscles in segments of the digestive tract that push the food onward.

**Peritoneum** is a lining (or two linings, actually): the **parietal** (which refers to a wall or partition) **peritoneum** lines the abdominal cavity; the **visceral** (which pertains to an organ) **peritoneum** covers the organs so is the inner lining of the two. The space between these two linings is the **peritoneal cavity**. You can perhaps deduce from this definition how serious **peritonitis** can be. The inflammation can easily spread throughout the entire abdomen.

**Stool** comes from usage as a seat with legs but no back or arms, then a toilet, then the waste expelled into that toilet. Quite a journey! The Greek combining form for the stool is **chez/o**, as in **hemat/o/chezia**, which tells us there is blood (**hemat/o**) in the stool. The Latin combining form is **fec/o** or **feces**. **Feces**, or *faeces* in Latin, means sediment or dregs.

A **sphincter** is a ring of muscles. The Greek verb *sphingein* means to bind tight or to squeeze. Do you see the word sphinx here? I refer you to the Greek myth of the Sphinx to read all about it. For now, it is enough to know that "Sphinx" means the Strangler! One example of a **sphincter** in the human body is the **pyloric sphincter**. This is the opening between the **stomach** and the **duodenum**. *Pyloros* is the Greek for gatekeeper, porter, or guard.

### Maladies and Unwellnesses

**A/chalasia:** The prefix **a-** means no, not, without, and **chalasia** is the condition of relaxing. Here, the muscles in the lower esophagus don't relax, thence food cannot enter the stomach. A former student sent me a story of her eighty-seven-year-old father, who suffered from this condition. He was treated with a series of Botox injections, which gave immediate but short-term relief. While on this regimen, he liked to tell his friends that he'd had Botox injections, but he neglected to tell them where he'd had the injections. His friends weren't sure why an eighty-seven-year-old needed Botox, and they couldn't see any cosmetic enhancement. Furthermore, why were these injections covered by insurance? It can be so much fun to stump one's friends once in a while!

**An/orex/ia:** The prefix **a-** or **an-** means no, not, without; the root **orex/i** means appetite, and the suffix **-ia** means condition. A lack of appetite. You may well have heard this word connected to **nervosa**. Another example is **orex/i/gen/ic,** pertaining to that which stimulates an appetite for food.

**Ascites** is a condition characterized by the abnormal accumulation of fluid in the peritoneal cavity; the abdomen becomes swollen or **distended**. The historical name for this condition is **dropsy**.

**Aphthous stomatitis** is a canker sore. **Aphth/o** is the combining form for ulcer, and **stomat/itis** is an inflammation involving the mouth.

**Borborygmus** is an example of onomatopoeia (a word that is a vocal imitation of the sound associated with it, such as buzz, fizz, or hiccup). **Borborygmus** is the gurgling, rumbling noises in the intestine caused by moving gas bubbles. It always seems to happen in a quiet setting with other people around, doesn't it?

**Diarrhea** and **dysentery** pertain to a looseness of the bowels. **Dysentery** was historically known as the bloody flux. It is an infection of the intestines marked by blood and mucus in loose stools.

The suffix **-emesis** has to do with vomiting, as in **hemat/ emesis,** which indicates blood in the vomit. An **emesis basin** is kept handy for—well, you know.

**Enema,** from the Greek meaning to send in or inject, is a procedure used to empty contents from the colon or for other therapeutic reasons including feeding, injecting drugs, anesthesia, or X-ray imaging.

An **eructation** is a belch or a burp.

**Hernia** is the Latin word for rupture. And that is what a hernia is sometimes called. It is the protrusion or bulging of an organ through whatever is containing it.

**Hiatal** comes from the Latin meaning an opening or gap. A **hiatal hernia** is the protrusion of the stomach upward through the esophageal hiatus (opening) in the diaphragm.

**Hyperphagia** is what a bear does just prior to hibernation. **Hyper/phag/ia** is the condition of eating an excessive amount. We might call it gluttony or binge eating in a human.

**Intussusception** is the inversion or telescoping of one portion of the intestine into another.

**Nausea** is from the Greek meaning seasickness. Do you see the family resemblance to the word "nautical"? To be **nauseated** or **nauseous** is to have the sensation that one may have to vomit. This is sometimes suffered after **hyper/phagia**.

**Obesity** comes from the Latin *obesitas,* meaning fatness or corpulence. And the Latin definition says it all.

**Orth/orex/ia nervosa** is an obsessive fixation with what one eats. Remember earlier we defined **an/orex/ia** as a condition of lacking an appetite? **Orth/o** means straight, and perhaps here it would help to think of it as straight and narrow, confined.

**Sial/o/aden/itis** is an inflammation of a salivary gland.

**Volvulus** is an obstruction caused by the twisting of the intestine onto itself.

Bon appetit!

# Chapter Ten
## The Urinary System

*"What is man, when you come to think about him, but a minutely set, ingenious machine for turning with infinite artfulness, the red wine of Shiraz into urine?"*
—Isak Dinesen (1885–1962)

Isak Dinesen is the *nom de plume* for Karen Blixen, a Danish writer. The movie *Out of Africa* was based on a portion of her life. Shiraz is one of the oldest cities of ancient Persia (modern-day Iran) known for producing the finest wine of the Middle East.

### Introduction

In days of yore, way back when amazing art was being painted on cave walls, urine and other bodily fluids such as blood and saliva were being used as material in the paints. By 4000 BCE, urine was a significant diagnostic tool. And sometimes a tool for prognostication. Color charts showing various shades of urine, from cloudy to red-tinged to amber, have been around a very long time.

For centuries, taste testing urine samples was an aid in diagnosis. Both ancient and present-day cultures have thought of the consumption of urine (**urophagia**) as a remedy, a cosmetic practice, or part of a health routine. Today, dogs can be trained to smell certain cancers in urine samples. Medical terms involving urine and the system that produces it are the subject of this chapter.

## Function

Why do we have a urinary system? Well, someone has to take out the garbage! True, the bottom end of the digestive system handles the solid waste management, but the urinary system takes care of waste products in the blood. Good at multi-tasking, this system also is involved with electrolyte balance (think sodium, potassium, calcium and such), blood pressure regulation, the management of red blood cell production, and the acid/base balance (**homeostasis**). The kidney is the primary organ, with supporting roles played by ureters, the urinary bladder, and the urethra.

## Key Vocabulary
## Kidney

There are two combining forms meaning kidney: **nephr/o** and **ren/o**. **Ren/o** is generally used in anatomic terms, while **nephr/o** is generally found in physiologic and clinical terms.

1. From the Greek comes **nephr/o**. Examples:
   **hydro/nephr/osis**   A condition (**-osis**) in which a kidney becomes swollen due to impaired drainage of urine. **Hydr/o** literally means water, as in "hydrant,"

"hydrate," or "hydroelectric," but can be used more generally to refer to a fluid.

**nephr/algia**   Refers to pain in a kidney.

**nephr/ectasia**   Distention or stretching of the kidney.

**nephr/o/ptosis**   A dropping, a displacement, of the kidney; the suffix **-ptosis** means dropping or drooping.

2. From Latin comes **ren/o**. Examples:

**reni/form**   Shaped like a kidney (as in a certain bean).

**ren/o/graphy**   Radiography (X-rays) of the kidney.

**ren/o/gastr/ic**   Pertaining to the kidney and stomach.

## Ureters

The **ureters** are two spaghetti-like tubes—one for each kidney—that transport the freshly made urine from the kidney to the urinary bladder.

## Urinary Bladder

The word **bladder** comes to us from the Anglo-Saxon *blaedre,* which refers to a blister or windbag. As with the combining forms for the kidney, the Greek combining form for the urinary bladder, **cyst/o**, is generally used in physiologic and clinical terms, while the Latin **vesic/o** is used in anatomic terms. "Generally" is the operative word in that last sentence.

1. Examples for **cyst/o**:

**cyst/o/rrhaphy**   Surgical suture of the urinary bladder.

**cyst/ectomy**   Surgical removal or resection of the urinary bladder.

**cyst/o/cele**   A herniated bladder.

2. Example for **vesic/o**:

> **vesic/o/clysis** A washing out, or lavage, of the urinary bladder. The suffix **-clysis** means lavage or wash; the word **lavage** comes from the Latin *lavatorium*, a place for washing. And now you know where the word "lavatory" comes from.

## Urethra

The urethra is the tube that empties the urinary bladder to the outside of the body. Now, if you find that you have a problem keeping the ureter and urethra untangled, here is a mnemonic that some students have used: There are two ureters and two *e*'s in ureter; there is only one urethra, spelled with only one *e*.

## Urine

The combining form is **ur/o** or **urin/o**, and the related suffix is **-uria**. The Latin source is *urina*. Examples:

> **ur/o/phag/ia** Pertaining to eating or swallowing urine; please note the comments in the introduction to this chapter.
>
> **urin/ation** The process of urinating; **-ation** means process or condition..
>
> **hemat/uria** Pertains to the presence of blood (**hemat/o**) in the urine.

There are more terms ending in **-uria** in the section on maladies below.

## Additional Vocabulary

**Fundus** is the Latin word for bottom or base. In the urinary bladder, it is the part closest to the rectum.

**Glomerul/o** is the self-evident combining form for the **glomeruli** (singular **glomerulus**), which are squiggly balls of capillaries that help filter the blood in the early stage of urine production. This term is from the Latin for a ball of yarn or thread, which gives a visual image of a glomerulus.

**Kegel exercises** are named for Arnold Kegel (1894-1981) and consist of alternately contracting and relaxing the pelvic floor muscles to improve urethral and rectal sphincter function. A sphincter is a ring of muscles such as is found in the rectum and the urinary meatus. Strong muscles help prevent leaking from urge or stress incontinence.

**Meat/o** is the combining form for **meatus,** which comes from the Latin *meare*, meaning go along, flow, travel. I am reminded of the word "meander." The **urinary meatus** forms a passage or opening from the bladder to the exterior of the body.

**Nephron** is the functional unit of the kidney and consists of a glomerulus and its accompanying tubule.

**Pyel/o** is the combining form for **pelvis;** in this case, the **renal pelvis**. It comes from the Greek for a tub-shaped vessel or basin. The Latin equivalent is **pelv/o**, used primarily in regards to the bony pelvis, which is also shaped like a basin. Examples:
> **pyel/o/nephr/itis** An inflammation of the **kidney** and the **renal pelvis**.

**pyel/o/gram**   An X-ray of the **renal pelvis** and other parts of the urinary system

**pyel/o/lith/o/tomy**   A surgical procedure in which an incision or opening is made (**-tomy**) in the renal pelvis (**pyel/o**) to remove a stone (**lith/o**).

**Urea** and **uric acid** are the primary waste products in **urine**. Don't confuse **urea** with the suffix **-uria**. They are homophones (**homo** means same and **phon/o** is sound).

Two related words for **urin/ation** are from the Latin, **mictur/ate** meaning to urinate, and **micturi/tion**, the condition or action of urination. To **void**, in this context, is to empty one's bladder.

### Maladies and Unwellnesses

**Catheter** is a word descended directly from the Greek *katheter* and means something inserted—which is what you do with any catheter. A urinary catheter is a tube inserted into the bladder to drain urine when it is not draining naturally, when there is **urinary retention**.

**Dialysis:** When the kidneys are not functioning effectively, this artificial process removes the waste and excess water from the blood.

**Enuresis** is the involuntary release of urine in one considered old enough to be "potty-trained." **Nocturnal enuresis** is the term for when these accidents occur at night—bed-wetting.

**Frequency** refers to urinating often, usually in small amounts; "going" frequently.

**Hypo/spadias/ epi/spadias/ para/spadias:** Sometimes in males the **urinary meatus** is found on the underside of the penis rather than in its usual location. This is **hypo/spadias. Epi/spadias** refers to it being found topside, and **para/spadias** indicates it is to one side. These are **congenital** (present at birth) conditions.

**Incontinence** refers to a person's inability to control the release of urine or feces. When we break this word down into its component parts, we get **in** (not), **con** (together), and **tin** (able to hold). In other words, not able to hold it together. **Stress incontinence** is transitory and can be caused by a sneeze or a cough, lifting a heavy object, or sometimes laughter. **Urge incontinence** is the leaking that occurs when the bladder is very full. It's time to do those Kegel exercises! (See above.) In another context, **incontinence** indicates the lack of control of sexual urges.

**Stones** can form in the kidney or the bladder. From the Greek we get the combining form **lith/o**, and from the Latin we get **calcul/o**. Just like the branch of mathematics known as calculus. The Latin word *calculus* means pebble (pebbles were once used in reckoning or counting). Here the pebble is made of mineral and acidic salts and is capable of causing great pain. The word for more than one pebble is **calculi. Nephr/o/lith/iasis** or **renal calculus** indicates a stone in a kidney and **cyst/o/lith/iasis** or **vesic/al calculus** in the bladder.

**-tripsy** is a suffix coming from the Greek *tripsis,* meaning friction or rubbing. I mention it here because **lith/o/tripsy** is a procedure using shock waves to break up, crush, and otherwise reduce to smithereens those nasty calculi. And no surgery is required.

**Turbid** is an adjective that describes milky or cloudy urine.

**Ur/emia** indicates the presence of urea (**ur**) in the blood (**emia**).

---

## -Uria

I've grouped some **-uria** ending words together.

In **an/uria,** the prefix **an-** indicates no, not, without, so this is a condition of being without urine. No urine is being produced by the kidneys.

**Bacteri/uria** pertains to the presence of bacteria in the urine.

**Dys/uria** takes a slightly different slant. It describes painful or difficult (**dys-**) urination—the process of urination, not the product (urine).

**Glycos/uria** and **glucos/uria** indicate the presence of an abnormal amount of sugar in the urine, which is commonly associated with diabetes mellitus. When taste-testing, early practitioners found the urine of certain individuals to be sweet to the taste. As a young child, I would hear adults speaking about someone having "sugar" which was short for "sugar diabetes."

**Hemat/uria** indicates the presence of blood in the urine.

**Noct/uria** is the term for frequently getting up to urinate at night (**noct/o**). Nocturia might indicate a medical condition, or it might mean you drank a lot of fluids before going to bed.

**Olig/uria:** The combining form **olig/o** means few or scanty. An "oligarchy" refers to a government, not of the people, but of a few people. In this medical condition, there is scanty urine output.

**Poly/uria** is the opposite of the above—**poly** means many—when the kidneys are busy and output is excessive.

**Py/uria Py/o** means pus so there's pus in the urine. A sign of an infection.

---

**Urgency** is a strong urge to urinate and a sense of pressure in the bladder as the bladder contracts repeatedly.

Congratulations! The final chapter awaits you.

# Chapter Eleven
## The Reproductive System

*"Wherever the art of medicine is loved, there also is love of humanity."*
—Hippocrates (c. 460–c. 370 BCE)

### Introduction

This is my favorite chapter. I can remember, as a senior student nurse, realizing that I had been through all the clinical rotations and the one I enjoyed the most was the birth room. Labor and delivery. I considered a career as a midwife. Years later, as a nurse recruiter, I had occasion to place ads in the local newspaper—that's what we did back then—for labor and delivery nurses. I received responses from truckers declaring they would labor and deliver! This is true. So, enjoy this chapter with me.

We will be considering the medical terms associated with the male and female reproductive systems, sexual intercourse, pregnancy, birth, and the newborn infant.

## Function

The title says it all. Human reproduction is about nothing less than assuring the survival of humankind. We will start with the gonads and the gametes.

## Female
## Key Vocabulary
## I Am Woman!

And these are the combining forms for female or woman: **gynec/o** as in **gynecology,** and **estr/a** or **estr/o** as in **estr/o/gen** or **estr/a/diol,** which is a steroid produced by the ovary.

### Female Gonads and Gametes

**Gonad** comes from the Greek *gone,* meaning seed. It is used here as the generic term for the sex organs: **ovaries** in the female and **testes** in the male. The sex organs or **gonads** produce the **gametes.**

**Gametes** are mature reproductive cells. In the female, the **ovaries** produce the **ova,** or eggs.

The **ovary** (plural **ovaries**) is the female **gonad.** The two combining forms are **ovari/o** and **oophor/o.**

1. **Ovari/o** is the combining form which comes from the Latin. Examples:
>    **ovari/o/rrhexis**    As the suffix **-rrhexis** refers to a rupture, so here the ovary has ruptured.
>    **ovari/ectomy** Surgical removal or resection of an ovary.

**ovari/o/cyesis**   An ectopic pregnancy in an ovary. The suffix **-cyesis** refers to a pregnancy, and the word **ectopic** comes from the Greek *ektopos*, meaning out of place.

2. **Oophor/o** is from the Greek. This combining form breaks down to **o/o**, which is the combining form for egg, and **phor**, meaning to bear or carry. So, bearing or carrying eggs is a function of the ovary, along with producing hormones. Examples:

**oophor/ectomy**   The surgical removal or resection of an ovary.

**oophor/o/cyst/ectomy**   The surgical removal or resection of an ovarian cyst.

**oophoroma**   A malignant ovarian tumor.

Eggs are the female **gamete**. In the Latin, **ovum** is one egg; **ova** refers to more than one egg. Ova are the biggest cells in the human body and can be seen with the naked eye. The combining forms are **ov/i** and **ovul/o**. Examples:

**ovi/cide**   A substance that kills (**-cide**) eggs.

**ovul/ation**   The ejection of a mature gamete/egg from the ovary.

The Greek combining form for the egg is **o/o** (as in the combining form **oophor/o** above). "Oval" is a common word and literally means pertaining to an egg.

**Oo/gene/sis** is the process by which the mature human **ovum** is formed, has its beginning (**genesis**). During the first three months of the female's embryonic life, the ovarian follicles develop. Then follow the processes of **mitosis** and then **meiosis**, which have to do with cell division.

At one point, the meiotic process is halted until this tiny embryonic female is born and grows to puberty. **Meiosis** resumes in the tiny developing **ovum** upon **ovulation**, but after further development stops again, only to complete the **meiotic** process and become the fully mature **ovum** upon fertilization.

### Anatomy—Internal

**Fallopian tubes** are the tubular **ov/i/ducts** from the **ovary** to the **uterus**. These tubes were named after Gabriele Falloppio (1523-62), an anatomist and physician. They are also called **ov/i/ducts**, as these tubes lead or provide a route for the eggs to the uterus. The word "duct" comes from the Latin infinitive *ducere*, which means to lead or guide. The word "viaduct," in which the Latin *via* means way, or "abduct," which means to lead away, from are common examples in English. The **Fallopian tubes** are also called **salpinges** (the singular is **salpinx**). This term comes from the Greek referring to a trumpet, and if you look at an image of this tube, I think you will see why. The combining form is **salping/o** as in **salping/o-oophor/ectomy**, a procedure in which the tubes and the ovaries have been removed surgically.

---

There are three combining forms for **uterus**: **uter/o**, **hyster/o**, and **metr/io** or **metr/o**.

1. The **uterus** or womb has the combining form **uter/o** from the Latin. Example:
    **uter/ine** Pertaining to the uterus.

From the Greek, there is **hyster/o** and **metri/o** or **metr/o**.

2. In Chapter One, when discussing the way meanings of words change over the years, I used the term **hyster/o** as an example. Perhaps you might want to refer to it now. Examples:

**hyster/ia**  Literally, a condition of the uterus; the story of how the meaning evolved is in the first chapter of this book.

**hyster/ectomy**  The surgical removal of the uterus.

**hyster/o/scopy**  The process of using an instrument (**hyster/o/scope**) to look inside and examine the uterus.

3. **Meter**, meaning measure, and **metri/o** or **metr/o** (uterus) are related. *Meter* is also a Greek word for mother as in the name Demeter, the mythological mother of Persephone. The woman's regular flow of blood, from no obvious wound, and which does not result in the death or weakening of the woman, was a profound mystery. Its regularity could provide a basis for the measurement of time. The menstrual time is still known as "moon time" and is a regular, natural, cyclic event. In a totally different setting, if you ride the metro you are referring back to the ancient roots of the mother city, the Greek *metropolis*. Example:

**my/o/metri/um**  The suffix **-um** means structure or thing, and **my/o** means muscle. This is the muscular wall of the **uterus**.

---

The **vagina** is the muscular tube or passage that leads from the **uterus** to the external **genitalia**, or the **vulva**. The **vagina** is also known as the birth canal in the context of pregnancy. The combining form **vagin/o** comes from the Latin; the Latin word *vagina* refers to a sheath or a scabbard. Another combining form for the vagina is **colp/o**. Examples:

> **vagin/o/myc/osis**    A condition (**-osis**) of fungus (**myc**) in the vagina.
>
> **colp/o/cleisis**    A surgical occlusion or closure of the vagina; the suffix **-cleisis** comes from the Greek signifying a closure.

### Anatomy—External

**Vulva** (**vulv/o** from the Latin and **episi/o** from the Greek) is the collective term for the female external genitalia, which include the **labia majora**, the **labia minora** (Latin for large and small lips respectively), the **clitoris**, the **vestibule** of the **vagina**, the **vaginal opening,** and the **Bartholin glands**. Examples:

> **vulv/o/vagin/itis**   An inflammation involving both the vulva and the vagina.
>
> **episi/o/tomy**    An incision made in the **perineum** during childbirth to aid in a difficult delivery and prevent the tearing of tissues.

**Perineum** with its combining form **perine/o** is the area between the vulva and the anus. Example:

> **colp/o/perine/o/rrhaphy**    The surgical repair of perineal and vaginal tears.

**Cervic/o** is the combining form for a **cervix** (plural **cervices**), which means neck. In the spine, this combining form refers to the **cervical vertebrae**; here, it refers to the **cervix** or neck of the **uterus**.

Another combining form for neck is **trachel/o** as in **trachel/ectomy**, the surgical removal of the uterine cervix.

## Additional Vocabulary

There are two combining forms for breast: **mast/o** and **mamm/o**.

1. **Mast/o** from the Greek *mastos.* Examples:
   **a/mast/ia**     The condition of a missing breast.
   **mast/ectomy**   The surgical removal or resection of a breast.
   **mast/o/ptosis** The suffix **-ptosis** (careful not to spit when you say this!) means to droop or sag. This can come with age. Carol Burnett used to say that she was now of the age where her bra size was a 34 long and her breasts were racing each other to her waist.

2. **Mamm/o** comes from the Latin *mamma.* Examples:
   **mamm/o/gram**   An image or X-ray of the breast.
   **mamm/o/plasty**   Surgical repair or reconstruction of a breast.

The small circular area around the nipple of the breast is the **areola**.

## Menstruation

**Men/o** is from the Latin *mensis*, the singular of **menses**, which means month. It refers to the monthly discharge of blood from the uterus, **menstruation**.

**Menstru/o** is the combining form for **menstruation**, the cyclic shedding of the uterine endometrium, which is discharged from the body as a bloody flow from the vagina.

**Menarche** has in it the Greek *arkhe,* meaning beginning— the beginning of the **menses**. A girl-child's first menses or moon time is the beginning of her womanhood. It is marked in a variety of ways by various cultures around the world.

**Menopause** is also sometimes called the climacteric or the "change of life". This marks the end of the menses and a woman's reproductive phase. Early on in my personal experience of this phenomenon, I had a dream in which I was sitting at my desk. In a drawer containing my hanging files I saw, as one only can in a dream, some embryos floating. Upon awakening, it came to me that from now on my offspring would be "brain child(ren)"—they would be the papers in hanging files, which now have evolved into files on my computer. This is the time of the crone, the wise woman, the elder.

**Mittelschmerz** is a one-sided abdominal pain coincident with **ovulation**. I know a woman who is sometimes aware of ovulating but says it isn't pain she feels, just a sense of awareness.

**Tubal ligation** is commonly referred to as "getting your tubes tied." The tubes referred to are the **Fallopian tubes,** and **ligation** comes from the Latin infinitive *ligare*, meaning to bind. This is a surgical procedure in which the tubes are cut and then tied, resulting in the inability of the woman to become pregnant.

## Maladies and Unwellnesses

The suffix **-atresia** breaks down to **-a/tres/ia** and indicates a condition of having no opening or perforation. The word part **tres** comes from the Greek *tresis*, meaning perforation. An example of this is **hyster/atresia**, which means the uterus has the abnormality of not having an opening.

**Dilation and curettage** (abbreviated frequently as **D/C**) is a surgical procedure in which the uterine cervix is dilated to accommodate a small curette, an instrument used for scraping the wall of the uterus. **Curettage** comes from the French meaning to clear or cleanse.

**Dys/par/eunia** signifies a difficult or painful intercourse. **Eunia** comes from the Greek meaning to go to bed or to lie alongside, while **dys-** means difficult or painful.

**Female genital mutilation** (**FGM**) is a partial or total removal of the vulva for non-medical reasons. A **clitorid/ectomy**, the surgical removal of the **clitoris**, has been associated in years past with cures for epilepsy, masturbation, and hysteria.

**Hormone replacement therapy** (**HRT**) is the use of hormones, usually **estrogen**, to treat the symptoms of **menopause** or osteoporosis.

---

## Menstrual Irregularities

**Dys/men/o/rrhea** refers to a difficult or painful flow or **mensis**.

**Meno/metro/rrhagia** indicates excessive bleeding during and between menstrual cycles.

**Meno/rrhagia** describes excessive bleeding during menstruation, sometimes referred to as flooding.

**Metro/rrhagia** is bleeding from the uterus at any time other than during normal menstruation (intermenstrual or non-menstrual bleeding).

**Metro/rrhea** indicates the discharge of mucus or pus from the uterus (even though you don't see the word part **py/o** or **muc/o**).

---

**Pre/menstru/al syndrome** is the term for the grouping of a wide variety of symptoms experienced by some women in the days immediately preceding the start of menstruation.

**Prolapse:** The suffix **-lapse** means slide so, **pro-** means a slide forward. (A slide backward would be a relapse.) In this chapter, **prolapse** would commonly be used to mean a **prolapsed uterus**.

**Py/o/salpinx** indicates the presence of pus in a **Fallopian tube**.

## Male
## Key Vocabulary
## Man Oh Man!

The combining form **andr/o** comes from the Greek *andro*, meaning man or male. As an example, android comes to mind, that which resembles (**-oid**) a man, or human in this case. The Latin-sourced combining form for male is **viril/o,** which immediately brings to mind the words "virile" and "virility." Examples:

**andr/o/pathy** A catch-all word that has to do with diseases unique to the male of the species, one of which is **prostatitis**.

**andr/o/pause** A collective word for physical and emotional changes that can occur as men age.

**andr/o/gyn/ous** Pertaining to having the characteristics of both the male and female (**gyn**).

## Male Gonads and Gametes

**Gonad** comes from the Greek *gone* meaning seed. We are using it as the generic term for the sex organs: the **testes** in the male and the **ovaries** in the female. The sex organs or **gonads** produce the **gametes**.

**Gametes** are mature reproductive cells. In the male, the **testes** produce the **spermatozoa**, often shortened to **sperm**.

**Testicle** and **testis** refer to the same **gonad**. The plural of **testis** is **testes.** Now, having established that, let's look at the combining form which comes to us from the Greek: **orch/o orchi/o** or **orchid/o.** If you see the name of a flower in there, you are on to something. Early anatomists noted a resemblance between the **testicle** and the fleshy tubers on the root-stocks of the orchid plant. Orchids have been used in traditional medicine to treat diseases. We will meet some medspeak examples using **orch/o** as we go along.

The Latin-based combining form also has an interesting story. **Test/o** or **testicul/o** comes from the Latin *testis,* which means witness. Some have said that this refers back to the days of Rome, when in a court of law men would take an oath with one hand resting on or covering their testes—swearing on their manhood, so to speak—that what they were about to say was true. (Today men and women can swear or affirm their veracity by raising their right hand.) Others dispute this connection. Related words are testimony, testament (as in last will and...), testify, contest, detest, and protest.

**Spermatozoa** or **sperm** are the **gametes**, the sex cells of the male. The average number of sperm that males produce varies but generally exceeds 100 million daily. My son-in-law's response to this production rate is, "Well, you can never say I just sit around all day doing nothing!" This is in stark contrast to the female, who is born with a lifetime of eggs—all she'll ever have—in her ovaries. I find this to be in parallel with the characteristics of masculine and feminine energies. Masculine energy, whether in the male or the female, is so of the moment, goal directed, decisive; feminine energy is much more about continuity, stability, relatedness. To be a whole, balanced person, we need to be conscious of and tap into both types of energy.

**Spermato/gene/sis** is the process by which sperm are produced. Here, as well as in the female, we find the processes of **mitosis** and **meiosis** in order to arrive at a mature sex cell.

**Semen** is a thickish, whitish fluid which contains **sperm** and liquids that help keep the fragile, tiny sperm alive. Do you know that the words "seminary" and "seminar" are from the same root as **semen**? The Latin *semen* means seed, and a *seminarium* is a seedbed or plant nursery.

The transporting tubules, providing a path for the sperm to and through the urethra of the male to the outside of the body, start with the **seminiferous** tubules, which are found in the testes and are the site of sperm cell production. The sperm next move into the **epididymis** (plural **epididymides**), which sit atop (**epi-**) the testes (**didymis**), and thence to the **vas deferens,** which in peristaltic waves moves the sperm along to the **urethra**.

Glands which contribute ingredients to semen include the **seminal vesicles,** which open into the **vas deferens**; the **prostate** (combining form **prostat/o**) **gland,** which "stands before " (from the Greek *prostates)* the urinary bladder to add the milky fluid to semen at the time of ejaculation; and the **bulboutethral** or **Cowper's gland.**

The external genitalia of the male include the **scrotum**, a sac of skin which holds the testicles, and the **penis**. The combining form for **penis** is **pen/o** from the Latin meaning tail. The penis provides a passage for both urine and semen to leave the body. **Balan/o** is the combining form for the **glans penis** which is the sensitive, rounded head of the penis. The Greek *balanos* means acorn.

### Additional Vocabulary

**Circumcision** in Latin means to cut (**-cision** as in incision) around (**circum** as in to circumnavigate the globe). In this case, it is the surgical removal of the foreskin or prepuce.

**Perineum,** with its combining form **perine/o**, is the area between the scrotum and the anus.

**Prepuce** is the term for the foreskin of the penis.

---

### Sexual intercourse

Many positions, many techniques, and many—well, a few—combining forms.

1. The Greek is **pareun/o** as in **dys/pareun/ia,** which is a painful or difficult sexual intercourse.

2. The Latin is **venere/o,** which traces back to Venus, goddess of love and beauty. An example is the word **venere/al.** Also from the Latin are **coit/o** as in **coit/us,** or sexual union, and **copulation** from the Latin *copulare,* meaning to join.

---

**Testosterone** is a sex hormone.

**Vas/ectomy** is the surgical excision of the vas deferens for the purpose of sterilization.

### Maladies and Unwellnesses

**A/sperm/ia** breaks down to the condition (**-ia**) of no (**a-**) sperm. **Olig/o/sperm/ia** is the condition of having few (**olig**) sperm. **A/zoo/sperm/ia** refers to the absence of live **spermatozoa** in the **semen.**

**Benign prostatic hyperplasia is** a common problem in men over fifty. It is a noncancerous enlargement of the prostate gland.

**Chancre** is a venereal ulcer. The word comes from the Latin *cancer*.

**Chlamydia** is a common bacteria-caused, sexually transmitted disease (STD); it is also known as non-gonococcal urethritis.

**Chordee** is a painful downward curvature of the penis during erection. It may be congenital (a birth defect).

**Crypt/orchid/ism** breaks down to a condition (**-ism**) of a hidden (**crypt**) testicle (**orchid**). Sometimes during fetal development, one or both testes fail to descend to the scrotum from the abdomen, where they begin their development. **Orchid/o/pexy** is the surgery which moves the wee testicle into the scrotum and surgically fixates it (**-pexy**). In non-medical usage, "crypt" refers to an underground room in a church often used for burials and hidden from view. A cryptonym is a hidden name, or a code name.

**Gender dys/phor/ia** applies to both the male and female and is the feeling (**phor**) that one's emotional and psychological being is at odds (**dys-**) with one's biological body.

**Gonorrhea** is an (STD) named for its primary symptom: urethral discharge. **Gono** means seed, and with the suffix **-rrhea** we have a flow or discharge of seed (semen as it was thought back then). An old slang term for gonorrhea is the clap. Females are also susceptible to this STD.

**Hemat/o/sperm/ia,** or the condition (**-ia**) of blood (**hemat/o**), does not really occur in the sperm but in the semen. This is uncommon and usually quite benign, going away on its own, but is also quite upsetting to the male experiencing it.

**Impotence** or **erectile dysfunction (ED)** is the chronic inability to attain or maintain an erection.

**Phimo/sis** is from the Greek *phimos,* meaning muzzle; it is the narrowing (**stenosis**) that precludes the foreskin from being drawn back over the glans penis.

**Priapism** derives from Priapus or Priapos, a minor, rustic, fertility god in Greek mythology. His legacy includes leaving his name to this condition in which there is an abnormally prolonged erection. The penis does not return to flaccidity.

**Vas/o/vas/ostomy** is the procedure which reverses the **vas/ectomy**.

**Varicocele** refers to the enlargement of a vein (a **varicosity**) in the scrotum.

### Infant
### Key Vocabulary

**Fertilization:** This section begins with the joining of a sperm and an egg: the fertilization of the egg. Usually this occurs within the body of a female, but there are instances in which it occurs **in vitro**. This term is Latin for "in glass" and refers to the petri dish in a laboratory. **Ecto/gene/sis** is a more general term that indicates a developing outside of the organism in which it would normally be found, such as in a "test tube baby." **To conceive** and **conception** are terms also applied to **fertilization**.

**Zygote** is the name given the fertilized egg. *Zygon* is Greek for yoke.

**Embryo:** The cells start to divide, rapid development occurs, and for the first eight weeks of this amazing journey, the new little being is called an **embryo.**

For the next thirty-two weeks of growth and change the term to know is **fetus**.

**Gestation** is the period between conception and birth; the carrying of young in the womb, **pregnancy**. These words are also used in situations such as "to be pregnant with possibility" and "to gestate ideas."

Another term for pregnancy, the combining form **gravid/o** or **gravidar/o** comes from the Latin *gravis,* meaning heavy or weighty, burdened. A **primi/gravida** refers to a first (**primi**) born. A closely related word is "gravitas," meaning authority or majesty. We sometimes hear the question: Does the candidate have the necessary gravitas to be president?

**Nat/o** is a combining form meaning birth. There are a variety of words in the English language which derive from this root. For instance, one's **natal** day is one's birthday. One is a native of a certain locale. But of one place only! I have read of someone about whom it was commented that "he is currently a native of Australia." His adopted country, perhaps, his current residence, perhaps, but his native land? Not unless he was born there!

Some familiar words in the context of human development are **pre/nat/al** (occurring before the birth), **post/nat/al** (occurring after the birth), **peri/nat/al** (occurring around, before or after, the birth event), and **neo/nat/al** (relating to the newborn).

**Obstetr/o** comes from the Latin for midwife. **Obstetr/ics** literally means the science of midwifery. In current usage, it refers to the care of a woman during childbirth.

**Para** comes from the Latin infinitive *parere*, meaning to bring forth. It is commonly used in the context of specifying the number of children a woman has delivered. **Primi/para** for a first-timer, **multi/para** for the experienced mother, and **nulli/para** for the woman who has never given birth. The prefix **nulli-** comes from the Latin *nullus* meaning no or none. To nullify something is to make it as nothing, to obliterate it. The word "annul" has always seemed like a redundancy to me: the prefix **an-** means no, not, without, and the word root **nul** means no or none! To annul a marriage is to declare it legally invalid or void. Another redundant expression we hear is "to make something null and void."

**Parturition** is the process, the action of giving birth. I remember this term by noting the word **part** within the term. The process of labor and birth is, indeed, a parting with the fetus the mother has carried for nine months. When

I was pregnant, I realized that this little being was closer to me than would ever be the case again. It was within my body, supported by my circulation, a part of me, yet not. However, before sonograms, I didn't even know the gender of this new one, let alone what physical features, personality preferences, etc., would be manifest. To learn all about this child, I would have to part with him/her. As parents know, this is only the first parting as our children grow and develop, hopefully becoming more and more their own healthy selves.

## Additional Vocabulary

In **amni/o/centesis,** the suffix **-centesis** has to do with a surgical puncture, often done to remove fluid for diagnostic assessment. In this case, the puncture is into the **amni/o/tic sac** and the fluid is **amni/o/tic fluid.** The **amnion** is the membranous sac enclosing the developing fetus. When one hears reference to waters breaking during a woman's labor, it is the membranes of the amnion which have ruptured, and the water is **amni/o/tic** fluid. Another example using this suffix is in a **thoracentesis,** when fluid is removed from between the lungs and the chest wall.

**Braxton Hicks contractions** have been called false labor, prodromal (running before—remember the reference to a dromedary camel in a previous chapter?), or practice contractions. They are the uterine muscles warming up, getting ready for the big event, pushing that baby out into the world. The name of the contractions is eponymous: John Braxton Hicks was a British physician.

**Colostrum** refers to the first secretions from the mammary glands as the breasts prepare for breastfeeding after the birth. Colostrum is loaded with protective antibodies for the newborn.

The **fontanel** is the area in the top of the infant's skull that is commonly referred to as the soft spot. The bones of the skull have not yet come together in the process called ossification. This is a neat design feature: not yet ossified, the bony plates can shift helping to ease the passage of the infant through the birth canal.

**Lactation**, from the combining form **lact/o**, refers to mother's milk. **Lactation** is the secretion of milk by the mammary glands. Related words are **lactic**, **lactose**, and **lactate**.

Now, that is the Latin. The Greek for milk is *galactos*. From this we get "galaxy," as in our very own home, the Milky Way, and **galact/ic**, pertaining to the flow of milk. The combining form is **galact/o.**

**Lightening** is the term used for the dropping of the baby into the position for a vaginal birth. It usually occurs about two to three weeks before the birth. Notice the difference in spelling between this and the "lightning" of an electrical storm.

**Meconium**, from the Greek *mekon,* meaning poppy, originally referred to the sap of unripe seed pods from the poppy flower. Along the way, anatomists began applying the term to the newborn's first bowel movement, which is greenish in color and consists of epithelial cells, mucus, and bile.

**Omphal/o** is the combining form for the belly button, the navel, the umbilicus.

**Omphaloskepsis** is the condition (**-sis**) of watching or observing the belly button, whether contemplating one's own navel as an aid to meditation or focusing on that of a belly dancer. James Kilpatrick, journalist, expressed his ecstatic love for words in the following excerpt from one of his columns: "Let us draw a beaded curtain over my affair with 'omphaloskepsis'. She was a belly dancer in a Cairo saloon. It was a brief affair. Enough!"

The word **umbilicus**—the navel or belly button—is related to the Latin *umbo* meaning the boss or protuberant part of a shield. It was used to designate either a raised or depressed spot in the middle of anything. An innie or an outie. It also refers to the cord, the **umbilical cord**, which connects the **fetus** to the mother's **placenta** in the **uterus**.

**Oxy/toc/ia** breaks down to **oxy** (rapid), **toc** (birth or labor), **ia** (condition): the condition of a rapid birth. An **oxy/toc/ic** is a labor inducing or accelerating drug. In other contexts **oxy,** as in "oxygen," means sour. "Oxygal" is an old word for sour milk.

**Placenta**, with the combining form **placent/o**, signifies the temporary organ in the uterus that provides nutrients to the developing little one through the umbilical cord.

**Puerper/o** comes from the Latin *puer,* meaning child, and *per,* meaning through. *Puer eternis* is a phrase used to mean a Peter Pan figure, one who "never grows up."

**Puerperal fever** used to be a quite common affliction for new mothers. Ignaz Semmelweis is a hero in the fight to get physicians to wash their hands when examining pregnant and delivering women. His story makes for a great read.

**Quickening** is the first time the mother feels the fetus move within her. Usually this occurs around gestational weeks eighteen to twenty.

### Maladies and Unwellnesses

The term **abortion** has different meanings for medical professionals and the general public. In general, it is thought of as specifically meaning the planned termination of a pregnancy. To medical professionals, the term has a broader meaning: a pregnancy has ended before a fetus is viable (able to live on its own). This general term can be modified to give more information. Examples:

**Spontaneous abortion**   An unplanned loss of a pregnancy, commonly called a miscarriage.

**Therapeutic abortion** The termination of a pregnancy for the health of the mother.

**Elective abortion**   The legal termination of a pregnancy for non-medical reasons.

**Eclampsia** is a complication of pregnancy marked by high blood pressure (**hypertension**) and convulsions, followed by coma and the threat of death. **Pre/eclampsia** is identified by hypertension, proteinuria, and edema (swelling). If not treated, eclampsia develops. **Puerperal eclampsia** is the term used when the convulsions occur immediately after the birth.

**Ectopic pregnancies** can occur in the ovaries and the abdominal cavity as well as the more common site, the fallopian tubes. Since 95 percent of ectopic pregnancies occur in the fallopian tubes, they are commonly called tubal pregnancies.

**Galactorrhea** refers to having too much of a good thing: after nursing has been discontinued, the milk continues to flow periodically.

**Gestational diabetes mellitus** is the development of diabetes during pregnancy in a woman who previously was not diabetic. Usually things return to normal after the birth, but care must be taken thereafter to avoid becoming diabetic.

**Hyperemesis gravidarum** is a severe form of the condition of early pregnancy commonly called "morning sickness." The name says a lot: **hyper** (excessive) and **emesis** (vomiting), while the **gravid** reminds us that this is occurring in a pregnancy. There is often weight loss and electrolyte imbalance creating the potential for a grave (**gravidarum**) situation.

**Mastitis** or inflammation of mammary glands: In years past, the term for this condition was milk fever.

**Placenta previa:** Think of something going before, previous, or **previa**. In this condition the placenta, instead of connecting to the top or side of the uterus, connects lower, occluding (closing off) part or all of the opening to the cervix. The placenta here is going before the fetus in the birth canal.

**Pseudo/cyesis** is a false (**pseudo**) pregnancy (**cyesis**). I saw this condition firsthand, not as a nurse, but with my father-in-law's little dachshund. Princess frequently developed that double row of nipples along her long underbelly without the benefit of male contact or the puppies.

You did it! This is the final chapter on a body system. I hope you enjoy the lighter verbal fare to come.

# Chapter Twelve
## Selection of Sundries

*"Health is a state of complete physical, mental, and social well-being and not merely the absence of disease or infirmity."*
—Preamble to the Constitution of the World Health Organization

The word **health** comes to us from the old English meaning wholeness; related words in the family tree of languages are the close relative "heal"; and there is "weal," meaning welfare or well-being, as in commonwealth, for the good of all; and also "holy" as in sacred.

**Disease** breaks down into the prefix **dis-,** which means to free of, to undo, separate, and **ease** is ease or comfort.

This segment contains a motley assortment of information that didn't make it into a specific chapter but deserves your attention.

**Malignant** and **benign** are two terms frequently heard in conversations about cancer. **Mal** connotes something negative, bad, even evil, while **bene** is good, well. The next component of the words, **ign,** comes from the Latin word *ignis,* which translates as fire. We use this regularly when we use the word "ignite." So, literally, we have bad fire and good fire. With regard to cancer, malignancies are known for their uncontrolled growth. Benign growths do not recur and do not metastasize. Other words with *mal* are malaise, malingerer, malicious, malpractice, malfunction. Some words on the positive side of the scale are benefit, beneficial, benefactor, benediction.

---

**On a lighter note,** a former student once told me that her five-year-old came to her and announced that he could not walk to school that day because his leg elbows hurt!

---

**Acute** and **chronic:** Perhaps you remember acute angles from math classes. The Latin word *acutus* means sharp or pointed. In a medical setting, where we might be talking about an acute pain, it indicates a coming and going quickly, brief but severe. **Chronic** comes from the Greek *chronos,* which means time, as in time measured by clocks, calendars, chronometers (a *chronos* measurer). Something chronic is linear, uniform, predictable. A chronology gives us the order in which things happened. Synchronized swimming tells us that things are happening at the same time, or together.

The Greeks had another word for time: *kairos.* It is more intuitive, organic, and what we mean when we say, "All in good time," "When the time is right," or "When things sort themselves out." We in the Western world are so into measured time these days, so clock conscious, so into instant or almost instant gratification, that we forget that there is another kind of time—when things are right.

---

**Etiology**, **diagnosis**, and **prognosis**:

**Etiology** is all about cause. It is the study of or the search for the cause of the disease or condition. In doing an etiologically oriented interview, questions will be asked about family history as there may be a genetic predisposition, or about environmental considerations, or work conditions. Is it bacteria causing the problem, or stress, or some other cause?

**Diagnosis** is about the signs and symptoms, the what-is-going-on. When we break down the word, starting with the suffix, **-sis** (condition or state of) and then the prefix **dia-** (complete, through) and finally the root **gno** (knowledge), we arrive at a definition: to know thoroughly. A diagnosis (plural **diagnoses**) results after a thorough, complete gathering of information, or knowledge, from all the tests, the patient interview(s), the observation of the clinicians, etc.

**Prognosis** is literally the condition (**-sis**) of prior (**pro-**) knowledge (**gno**). We use this term today in the same way Hippocrates did in ancient Greece, meaning to foretell the course of a disease.

A note on *gnosis*: a condition (**-sis**) of knowledge (**gno**). There was a group of people known as the Gnostics who lived in the Middle East at the same time as the early Christians. Without going into their beliefs, I will just call attention to the fact that there are still today those who call themselves agnostics, where the prefix **a-** means no, not, without.

---

**Pathology** comes from the Greek word *pathos*, which indicates suffering, feeling, emotion. In medical terminology, it has come to mean disease. Thence, **path/o/logy** is the study of disease and disease processes. Some non-medical words deriving from *pathos* that may be familiar are: apathy, pathetic, sympathy, and empathy.

---

**Iatr/o** is a combining form that derives from the Greek *iatros* meaning physician. It has come to mean «to treat." Some words in which we find this root are: **ped/iatr/ic**, **psych/iatr/y**, and **iatr/o/gen/ic**. This last word may be unfamiliar to you. The suffix (**-ic**) means pertaining to. There are two roots: **iatr/o**, which means treatment, and **gen**, which refers to formation, cause, to produce, and source. Pertaining to having its source in the treatment. Or, to put it another way: in the process of a treatment regimen, the person experiences a negative effect. Examples may help to clarify this: an EMT is expertly doing CPR and fractures the person's rib; a Foley catheter inserted into a urinary bladder results in an infection; in the process of receiving chemotherapy treatments, a person loses their hair.

**Nosocomial**: **Nos/o** is disease and -comial is from the Greek meaning "I take care of." The meaning of this word overlaps with **iatrogenic** in that a **nosocomial** infection is acquired in a hospital where one has gone to be treated or healed.

**Idi/o** is a combining form signifying the person or self. An **idi/o/path/ic** disease is of unknown cause or is unique to the person. This also applies to drug reactions: an **idi/o/path/ic** response to a medication is one that has not been observed in the general population. The word "idiolect" refers to the speech habits peculiar to a particular person. Since the source of **idi/o** is in the Greek *idios*, which means own or private, perhaps an idiot is someone who simply marches to their own drum ... or does their own thing.

## Pertaining to Suffixes

There are a number of suffixes that pertain to "pertaining to." Here is a list with examples:

**-ac** as in celiac
**-al** as in inguinal
**-an** as in caesarian
**-ar** as in plantar fasciitis
**-ary** as in maxillary
**-eal** as in ischeal, galacteal
**-iac** as in hemophiliac
**-ic** as in acoustic
**-ical** as in psychological
**-ine** as in iodine
**-ior** as in posterior
**-ose** as in glucose
**-ous** as in cutaneous
**-tic** as in neurotic

One of my former students told me that while she was studying flash cards, her eleven-year-old expressed curiosity about what she was doing. So, she went over some of the terms with him. A while later he came to her with a pained expression on his face and the explanation that his friend had kicked him in the "inguin"! Ouch!!

## Look Alikes But Not Alike

**ante-** Before as in ante meridian (a.m.), before the middle of the day, or ante cibum (a.c.), a common medication instruction for before meals.

**anti-** Against as in anti-coagulants.

**melatonin** A hormone secreted by the pineal gland.
**melanin** A pigment that gives skin, hair, and eyes their color.

**palpate** To examine parts of the body by touch.
**palpitate** A rapid, strong, perhaps irregular beating of the heart.

**ileum** A portion of the small intestine.
**ilium** Part of the pelvis.

**mucus** is the noun.
**mucous** is the adjective.

**hidr/o** Sweat.
**hydr/o** Water.

**mitosis**   A type of cell division.
**miosis**   Abnormal contractions of the pupil in the eye.

**oral**   Has to do with the mouth.
**aural**   Has to do with the ear.

**malleus**   One of the small bones in the inner ear.
**malleolus**   A hammer-shaped projection from a bone.

**my/o**   Combining form for muscle.
**myc/o**   Combining form for fungus.
**myel/o**   Combining form for both the spinal cord and bone marrow.

**py/o**   Combining form for pus.
**pyr/o**   Combining form for fever or for fire (think Pyrex).
**pyel/o**   Combining form for the renal pelvis.

**palliative**   To make something more bearable, less painful. It may be a dose of a narcotic or as simple as a cool washcloth on the brow. It is used particularly when a medical condition is without cure and one strives to make the person comfortable.

**placebo**   An inert pill, sometimes called a "sugar pill," or something done which has no therapeutic effect. A placebo may be used within the control group of a research experiment or perhaps simply to calm or to please a person. Interestingly, *placebo* is Latin for "I shall please."

**panacea**   A hypothetical cure-all, a universal remedy, or magic bullet that will take care of all your problems. Panacea is the name of the Greek goddess of healing.

---

It could have been a contemporary of ours, but it was Hippocrates who said that "walking is man's best medicine."

---

## The Colors of Medicine

**Albin/o** (from the Latin) . . . . . white
**Leuk/o** (from the Greek) . . . . . white
**Anthrac/o** . . . . . . . . . . . . . . . . black
**Melan/o** . . . . . . . . . . . . . . . . . black
**Chlor/o** . . . . . . . . . . . . . . . . green
**Cirrh/o** . . . . . . . . . . . tawny yellow
**Jaund/o** . . . . . . . . . . . . . . yellow
**Lute/o** . . . . . . . . . . . . . . . . yellow
**Xanth/o** . . . . . . . . . . . . . . . yellow
**Poli/o** . . . . . . . . . . . . . . . . . . gray
**Cyan/o** . . . . . . . . . . . . . . . . . blue
**Eosin/o** . . . . . . . . . . . . . . . . rosy
**Erythr/o** . . . . . . . . . . . . . . . . red

(**Eosin/o** gets its name from Eos, a Titaness and the goddess of the rosy dawn. Her Roman counterpart is Aurora, as in the Aurora Borealis and Aurora Australis.)

---

## Three Suffix Groupings

### 1. The double *rr*'s
    **-rrhaphy**  Suture.
    **-rrhea**     Flow, discharge.
    **-rrhexis**   Rupture.

**-rrhage** or **-rrhagia**     From the Greek *rhegnynai*, which translates to burst forth; it is excessive, profuse flow compared to **-rrhea** as in hemorrhage.

## 2. Meet the *-tomy*'s

**-ectomy** To remove, excise (ex/cise or, to cut from), resection.

**-tomy**     The process of cutting (**tom/o** is to cut).

**-tome**     An instrument used for cutting.

**-stomy** The process of forming a new mouth or opening (**stoma**).

If one performs a **trache/o/tomy**, one cuts into the trachea. If one used the suffix **-ectomy,** one would be removing all or part of the trachea. If a **trache/o/stomy** were performed, one would be more than cutting into the trachea— one would be creating a more "permanent" opening for someone who will need the opening indefinitely. The same with colostomy. A **colotomy** opens or makes an incision into the colon. The **colostomy** is indefinite and requires a colostomy bag and much dermal care. **Stomat/o** and **os** mean mouth.

## 3. Further Developments

All these suffixes have to do with development, formation, producing, causing:

**-blast**     Embryonic, immature.

**-trophy**     Development, nourishment.

**-poiesis**  Formation, development.

**-plasia**     Formation, growth.

**-genesis**  Producing, forming.

# Epilogue

Over the years, I have come across some picturesque, homey, even lovable words that say that one is not feeling so well. I don't want them to become obsolete, so I offer these five to you.

**Collywobbles**   To complain of the collywobbles is to have a bellyache or that feeling of queasiness in the tummy.

**Discombobulated**   To be disconcerted or confused, or perhaps upset or frustrated.

**Mubble fubbles**   A state of depression, or melancholy; despondency, low spirits.

**Mulligrubs**   A state of low spirits, the blues; grumpy.

**Peely-wally**   To look pale, sickly, wan, perhaps a bit feeble; as in "You look a bit peely-wally this morning. Are you sure you're not coming down with something?"

# Many Gratitudes

My heart is full of gratitude for the many contributions of so many people who have brought this book to publication.

Donna Frownfelter, at some point during those life-changing days as students at Loyola University Chicago, you planted the seed in my mind that teaching materials can be developed into a book.

Bruce Wingerd, I used your text, "Unlocking Medical Terminology" from the time it was first published through to my retirement from teaching. This convinced me never to write a textbook; I would never compete with yours.

Students in my "Introduction to Medical Vocabulary" course who asked if I had ever considered writing a book and encouraged me to do so, you nurtured the seedling/embryo of this brainchild.

Beta readers, namely: April and Donovan Malley, Gail and Chuck Painter, Tom and Priscilla Tepe, Steven Thomas, Matt Urbanski, and Shelly Waram, you were asked to perform the role of beta reader for me because I knew the variety of perspectives and skills that you would bring to this work. Perhaps more importantly, I knew that you would give me honest feedback. Thank you for sending me pretty much back to square one. But, at the same time assuring me that there was "something here" to work on and that I should not give up. You freely shared of your gifts and skills. Your patience, support and encouragement are valued beyond price.

The staff at Renton Dental Arts, led by Dannette Hooper, you suggested the list of words to include in the vocabulary of dentistry section. Your excellence in this contribution, in your professional work and your exceptional office culture have me singing your praises.

Stephanie Lawyer, your appearance in my life was synchronicity. Thank you for applying your professional copyediting skills to my little book. I will always associate cups of tea and good conversation with our business meetings at the Nordstrom Grill.

Epigraph Publishing Service, we met online and I fell in love with the content of your website. All those good reviews didn't hurt either. Thank you for taking on this neophyte author. May your days be long, healthy and profitable.

Lastly, to all of you who, when we meet at the market, or wherever, stop and ask me how my book is going, you have helped me believe that this book/brainchild just might be born. With your encouragement I have transitioned into an author, ready to acknowledge that I feel another book or two gestating inside me.

# Index

The medical terms and word parts found in this book are listed below in alphabetical order along with the chapter in which they can be found.

allurophobia - 6
alopecia - 2
alveoli - 8
alveol/o - 8
amastia - 11
ambidextrous - 7
amnesia - 1, 6
amniocentesis - 11
amnion - 11
amputation - 3
anabolism - 9
anacusis - 7
anal - 9
analgesia - 6
anaphylaxis - 4
anapnea - 8
andr/o - 5, 11
androgen - 5
androgynous - 11
andropathy - 11
andropause - 11
androphobia - 6
anechoic - 4
anemia - 4
anencephalography - 6
anencephaly - 6
anesthesia - 6
aneurysm - 4, 6
angina - 1, 4
angi/o - 4
angiocardiopathy - 4
angioplasty - 4
anhidrosis - 2

anisocoria - 7
ankyl/o - 3
ankylosis - 3
anorexia - 9
anosmia - 7
anoxic - 8
antagonism - 5
antecubital - 2
anthro - 4
antibiotics - 4
antibody - 4
anticoagulant - 4
antigen - 4
antigingivitis - 9
anti-pruritic - 2
antitoxins - 4
anxiolytic - 4
an/o - 9
anuria - 10
anus - 9
aorta - 4
aort/o - 4
apex - 4, 9
aphakia - 7
aphagia - 6
aphasia - 6
aphth/o - 9
aphthous - 9
apical - 4
apnea - 8
apoplexy - 1, 4, 6
appendix - 9
apraxia - 6

## B

bile - 9
bil/i - 9
binocular - 7
bipolar - 6
blephar/o - 7
blepharoptosis - 7
blepharospasm - 7
blood pressure - 4
bolus - 9
borborygmus - 9
bowel - 9
brachiate - 3
brachi/o - 3
brachydactyly - 3
bradycardia - 4
bradykinesia - 3
bradypnea - 8
brain - 6
bronchiole - 8
bronchoscope - 4
bronchus - 8
bruxism - 9
buccal - 9
bulbourethral - 11
bulla - 2
bursa - 3
bursectomy - 3
bursitis - 3
bursolith - 3

C

calc/i - 1

calcipenia - 1, 5
calcul/o - 10
calculus - 3, 10
capillary - 4
capn/o - 8
caput - 3
carbuncle - 2
carcin/o - 2
carcinogenic - 2
carcinoma - 4
card/o - 4
cardi/o - 1, 4
cardiology - 1
cardiomegaly - 4
cardiomyopathy - 4
cardiomyopexy - 4
cardiovascular accident - 4
caries - 9
carotid - 4
carpal - 3
carp/o - 3
cartilage - 3
cartilaginification - 3
cartilaginous - 3
cartilag/o - 3
catabolism - 9
cataract - 7
catarrh - 8
catharsis - 9
catheter - 10
cauda equina - 6
causalgia - 6
caus/o - 6

conjunctiva - 7
conjunctivitis - 7
conscious - 6
contusion - 2
convulsion - 6
convuls/o - 6
copulation - 11
corium - 2
corneal - 7
corne/o - 7
corneoblepharon - 7
cor/o - 7
coronary - 4
coron/o - 4
coronoid - 4
cortex - 5
coryza - 8
cost/o - 3
costectomy - 3
cranial - 3, 6
crani/o - 3
cranium - 3
cran/o - 3
crepitation - 3
cretinism - 5
crin/o - 5
croup - 8
crypt/o - 2
cryptorchidism - 11
curettage - 11
cusp - 4
cutane/o - 2
cutaneous - 2

cyan/o - 2
cyanosis - 2, 4
cyesis - 11
cynophobia - 6
cyst - 2, 10, 11
cystectomy - 10
cyst/o - 10
cystocele - 10
cystolithiasis - 10
cystorrhaphy - 10
cyt/o - 4

D

dacry/o - 7
dacryoadenalgia - 7
dacryohemorrhea - 7
dacryostenosis - 7
dactyl/o - 3
debride - 2
debridement - 2
decubitus - 2
defecation - 9
defibrillator - 4
deglutition - 9
delusions - 6
dementia - 6
dendrites - 6
dent/i - 9
dentifrice - 9
dentin - 9
dentist - 9
depilatory - 2

epidemic - 8
epidermomycosis - 2
epididymis - 11
epiglottis - 8
epiglott/o - 8
epileps/o - 6
epilepsy - 1, 6
episi/o - 11
episiotomy - 11
epispadias - 10
epistaxis - 8
eponychium - 2
erector - 3
eructation - 9
erythema - 2
erythrocytopenia - 4
erythr/o - 2, 4
erysipelas - 2
erythroderma - 2
esophag/o - 1, 9
esophagogastroduodenos-
copy - 1
esophagus - 9
esthes/o - 6
esthetician - 6, 9
esthetics - 6
estr/a - 11
estradiol - 11
estr/o - 11
estrogen - 5, 11
ethm/o - 3
ethmoid - 3
eugenics - 8

eupepsia - 9
eupnea - 8
eustachian - 7
euthanasia - 1, 8
euthyroid - 8
euthyroidism - 5
excoriate - 2
exhale - 8
exocrine - 2, 5
exophthalmos - 5
exoskeleton - 3
expectorant - 8
expire - 8

## F

fallopian - 7, 11
fasting blood sugar - 5
feces - 9
fec/o - 9
female genital mutilation - 11
femoris - 3
fer - 2
fertilization - 11
fetus - 11
fibrillation - 4
fibr/o - 2
fibrous - 2
fontanal - 11
frequency - 10
fundus - 10
furuncle - 2

# G

galactic - 11
galact/o - 11
galactorrhea - 11
gall - 9
gamete - 7, 11
gamophobia - 6
ganglion - 6
gastr/o - 1, 9
gastroenterocolitis - 9
gastroenterologist - 9
gastroenterology - 1
gastroesophageal - 9
gastrointestinal - 9
gastroscope - 9
genitalia - 1
gestation - 11
gingiv/o - 9
glands - 5
glans penis - 11
glaucoma - 7
glia - 6
glomerul/o - 10
glomerulous - 10
gloss/o - 9
glossolalia - 9
glossoplegia - 9
glossotrichia - 9
glottis - 8
glucose - 5
glucosuria - 10
gluteus maximus - 3

glycosuria - 10
gnath/o - 9
goiter - 5
gonad - 5, 11
gonorrhea - 11
grand mal - 6
gravidar/o - 11
gravidarum - 11
gravid/o - 11
grippe - 8
gustation - 9
gynec/o - 11
gynecology - 11
gynephobia - 6
gyrus - 6

# H

halitosis - 8
hal/o - 8
hallucinate - 6
heart - 4
hematemesis - 9
hemat/o - 4, 9, 10, 11
hematochezia - 4, 9
hematology - 3, 4
hematophilia - 4
hematopoiesis - 3, 4
hematospermia - 11
hematuria - 10
hemiplegia - 3
hem/o - 4, 7
hemoglobin A1c - 5

hemolysis - 4
hemophobia - 6
hemoptysis - 8
hemorrhage - 4, 6
hemorrhoids - 9
hemostasis - 4
hemostat - 4
hernia - 9
herpes zoster - 4, 6
heter/o - 2
heterograft - 2
hiatal - 9
hidr/o - 2
hidradenitis - 2
hirsutism - 2, 5
hirsut/o - 2
homeostasis - 4
homo - 2
homograft - 2
hordeolum - 7
hormone - 5, 11
humors - 4
hydr/o - 6, 10
hydrocephalus - 6
hydronephrosis - 10
hygiene - 1
hyoid - 3
hyperacusis - 7
hypercapnia - 8
hyperemesis - 11
hyperhidrosis - 2
hyperkalemia - 5
hyperopia - 7

hyperphagia - 9
hyperpnea - 8
hypersecretion - 5
hyperthyroidism - 5
hyperventilate - 8
hypnosis - 1
hypocalcemia - 5
hypochondria - 1
hypodermic - 2
hypokalemia - 5
hypophysis - 5
hyposecretion - 5
hypospadias - 10
hypothalamus - 5
hypothyroidism - 5
hypoxic - 8
hysteratresia - 11
hysterectomy - 11
hysteria - 1, 11
hyster/o - 1, 11
hysteroscope - 11
hysteroscopy - 11

I

iatr/o - 6
ichthy/o - 2
ichthyosis - 2
icterus - 2
ileum - 9
ilium - 9
immune - 4
impotence - 11

larynx - 8
laxative - 9
lei/o - 2
leiodermia - 2
lenticular - 7
lenticul/o - 7
lent/o - 7
lentopathy - 7
leukemia - 2
leuk/o - 2
leukocytes - 2
leukoderma - 2
ligament - 3
ligation - 11
lightening - 11
lingual - 9
lingu/o - 9
linguogingival - 9
lipids - 2
lip/o - 2, 9
liposuction - 2, 9
lith/o - 3, 9, 10
lithotripsy - 10
lord/o - 3
lordosis - 3
lunula - 3
lymph - 4
lymphadenitis - 4
lymphocytes - 4
lymphoid - 4

**M**

macrophage - 4
macrophagocyte - 4
macrothrombocytopenia - 1
macula - 7
macular degeneration - 7
macule - 2
malignancy - 4
malleus - 7
malodorous - 7
mamm/o - 11
mammogram - 11
mammoplasty - 11
mandible - 9
mastectomy - 11
mastication - 9
mastitis - 11
mast/o - 3, 11
mastoptosis - 11
mastoid - 3, 7
maxilla - 9
meat/o - 10
meatus - 10
meconium - 11
medulla - 5
meibomian - 7
meiosis - 7, 11
melanin - 2
melan/o - 2
melanocytes - 2
melanoma - 2
melatonin - 5

## N

neonatal - 11
nephralgia - 10
nephrectasia - 10
nephr/o - 10
nephrolithiasis - 10
nephron - 10
nervosa - 9
neuralgia- 6
neurectasia - 6
neur/o - 6
neuroclonic - 6
neurodegenerative - 6
neuroglial - 6
neuron - 6
neuropathy - 6
neuroplasticity - 6
neurotransmitter - 6
noct/o - 10
nocturia - 10
node - 4
nodule - 2
nostril - 8
nucha - 3
nullipara - 11
nyctalopia - 7

# O

obesity - 9
obstetrics - 11
obstetr/o - 11
occlusal - 9
ochlophobia - 6

ocularist - 7
ocul/o - 7
oculus dexter - 7
oculus sinister - 7
oculus uterque - 7
odont/o - 9
olfaction - 7
olig/o - 10, 11
oligospermia - 11
oliguria - 10
om/o - 3
omphal/o - 11
omphaloskepsis - 11
onychectomy - 2
onych/o - 2
onychocryptosis - 2
onychomalacia - 2
onychomycosis - 2
onychophagia - 2
o/o - 11
oogenesis - 11
oophorcystectomy - 11
oophorectomy - 11
oophor/o - 11
oophoroma - 11
ophthalmia - 1
ophthalm/o - 7
ophthalmology - 7
ophthalmoplegia - 7
ophthalmoscope - 7
opsimath - 6
optician - 7
opticokinetic - 7

# P

pachyderm - 2
pachyderma - 2
pachy/o - 2
palatal - 9
palpation - 4
palpebrate - 7
palpebr/o - 7
palpitation - 4
palsy - 6
panacea - 1
pancreas - 5, 9
papule - 2
para - 11
paranoia - 6
paraplegia - 3
parasomnia - 6
paraspadias - 10
parathyroid - 5
paresthesia - 6
pareun/o - 11
parietal - 4, 6, 8, 9
parotid - 7
parotitis - 7
parturition - 11
patella - 3
pathogen - 4
pectoral - 8
pector/o - 8
pedicul/o - 2
pediculosis - 2
ped/o - 3

pellagra - 2
pelv/o - 10
penis - 11
pen/o - 11
peps/o - 9
pept/o - 9
pericardium - 1, 4
perinatal - 11
perine/o - 11
perineum - 11
periodontal - 9
periosteum - 3
peristalsis - 9
peritoneum - 9
peritonitis - 9
pertussis - 8
petechiae - 2
petit mal - 6
phac/o - 7
phacopathy - 7
phag/o - 2, 4
phagocytosis - 4
phak/o - 7
phakoma - 7
phalanges - 3
pharyngitis - 8
pharyng/o - 8
pharyngotomy - 8
pharynx - 7, 8
pharmacist - 4
phimosis - 11
phlebitis - 4
phleb/o - 4

prostat/o - 1, 11
pruritus - 2
pseudocyesis - 11
psoriasis - 2
psychiatry - 6
psych/o - 6
psychosis - 6
psychosomatic - 6
psychotherapy - 6
pterygium = 7
ptysis - 8
puerperal - 11
puerper/o - 11
pulmonary - 4, 8
pulmon/o - 8
pulse - 4
pupil - 7
pupill/o - 7
purpura - 2
purulent - 2, 8
purul/o - 8
pustules - 2
pyel/o - 10
pyelogram - 10
pyelolithotomy - 10
pyelonephritis - 10
pyloric - 9
py/o - 2, 7, 8, 10, 11
pyorrhea - 2
pyosalpinx -11
pyothorax - 8
pyuria - 10

**Q**

quadriceps - 3
quadriplegic - 3
quickening - 11

**R**

radic/o - 6
radiculitis - 6
radicul/o - 6
radiculopathy - 6
radius - 4
rectalgia - 9
rectum - 3, 9
rectus - 3
renal - 10
reniform - 10
ren/o - 10
renogastric - 10
renography - 10
respiration - 8
resuscitate - 8
rhinitis - 8
rhin/o - 7, 8
rhinoplasty - 7
rhinorrhea - 8
rhinotillexis - 8
rhiz/o - 6
rhizotomy - 6
rhytidectomy - 2
rhytid/o - 2
rhytidoplasty - 2

rods - 7

**S**

salivary - 9
saliv/o - 9
salpinges - 11
salping/o - 7, 11
salpingo-oophorectomy - 11
sarc/o - 2
sarcoidosis - 2
sarcolysis - 2
schizophrenia - 6
sclera - 7
scler/o - 2
scleroderma - 2
sclerosis - 4
scoli/o - 3
scoliosis - 3
scrotum - 11
sebace/o - 2
sebaceous - 2
seb/o - 2
sella turcica - 3, 5
semen - 11
seminal vesicles - 11
seminiferous - 11
sepsis - 4
seps/o - 2
septic - 2
septicemia - 4
septum - 4, 8
serum - 4

shingles - 6
sial/o - 9
sialoadenitis - 9
sialoadenotomy - 9
sialolith - 9
sigmoid - 3, 9
sinus - 8
sinus/o - 8
skeleton - 3
somat/o - 6
somatic - 6
somnambulate - 6
somniloquy - 6
somn/o - 6
sperm - 11
spermatogenesis - 11
spermatozoa - 11
sphen/o - 3
sphenoid - 3
sphincter - 9
sphygm/o - 4
sphygmomanometer - 4
spir/o - 8
splenomegaly - 4
spondyl/o - 3
spondylolisthesis - 3
spontaneous - 8
sputum - 8
stapes - 7
steat/o - 2, 9
steatopygia - 9
steatorrhea - 2
stenosis - 4, 11

## SUFFIXES

-emia - 2, 4, 5, 10

-eunia - 11

-form - 2, 3, 7, 10

-gen - 2, 5, 11

-genic - 1

-gram - 4, 10, 11

-graphy - 6, 10

-ia - 1, 3, 4, 5, 6, 7, 8, 9, 10, 11

-ic - 2, 4, 6, 7, 8, 9, 10, 11

-ician - 6, 7, 9

-icle - 3, 7, 11

-in - 10

-ion - 3, 7, 8, 9

-ism - 2, 5, 6, 7, 9, 11

-ist - 4, 7, 9

-itis - 1, 2, 3, 4, 5, 6, 7, 8, 9, 10, 11

-ium - 2

-lapse - 11

-logist - 2, 4, 9

-logy - 1, 2, 4, 7, 11

-lysis - 2, 3, 4

-malacia - 2, 3, 9

-meter - 4, 7

-megaly - 2, 4, 5

-oid - 2, 3, 4, 5, 6, 7, 8, 9, 11

-ole - 5

-oma - 2, 3, 4, 7, 9, 11

-opia - 7

-opsia - 7

-ose - 2, 7

-osis - 2, 3, 4, 6, 7, 8, 10, 11

-ous - 2, 3, 4, 5, 7, 9, 11

-oxia - 5

-pathy - 1, 2, 4, 6, 7, 11

-penia - 4, 5

-pexy - 4, 11

-phagia - 2, 5

-phasia - 3, 6

-phil - 4

-phobia - 2, 3, 6, 7

-phragm - 4, 8

-phyte - 3

-plasia - 3, 5, 11

-plasticity - 6

-plasty - 1, 2, 3, 4, 7, 11

-plegia - 3, 7

-pnea - 8

-poiesis - 4

-ptosis - 7, 11

-rrhage - 4, 6

-rrhagia - 11

-rrhaphy - 3, 9, 10, 11

-rrhea - 2, 5, 7, 11

-rrhexis - 11

-scope - 4, 7, 9, 11

-scopy - 1, 2, 3, 11

-sis - 2, 5, 7, 11

-stasis - 4, 9

-stenosis - 7

-stomy - 8

-tic - 6

-tillexis - 5

-tome - 3

-tomy - 1, 6, 7, 8, 9, 10, 11

CPSIA information can be obtained
at www.ICGtesting.com
Printed in the USA
FSOW01n2359250716
22960FS